MEDICINE IN THE BACK OF BEYOND

ALSO BY DR. ROBERT C. EELKEMA

(with Tom Clifford and Patrick A. McGuire)

Good Medicine: *How Wit and Guile Saved the School of Medicine at the University of North Dakota*

Forty years ago, the
difficulty of recruiting doctors
to sparsely populated rural areas
left vast stretches of countryside
without any medical care at all...

Medicine in the Back of Beyond

Robert C. Eelkema, D.V.M., M.D., M.P.H.
with Patrick A. McGuire

How a savvy North Dakota public health doctor helped pioneer a radical strategy that extended the reach of doctors into rural America.

To Mark Pendergast — always engaged & on writing Warm regards
Robert Eelkema
5/21/13

Published by Dr. Robert C. Eelkema
Grand Forks, ND

Library of Congress Control Number: 2012906626
ISBN: 978-0-9854734-0-2

2 4 6 8 10 9 7 5 3 1

Printed by Cushing-Malloy, Inc.
Ann Arbor, MI

Illustrations by Arlene Feist
Edited by Pamela D. Knudson
Cover and interior book design by Gary Niemeier

Dedication

In 1974 in the volume "New Health Practitioners," published by the National Institutes of Health, I wrote the following:

> *"If the world were ideal, we would rub the magic lamp and the genie would grant our every wish. But what is the ideal in terms of the health care system? It is easy access, easy ingress, excellent education, ideal treatment and perfect results—a healthy mind, body and soul. Unfortunately the demand for this ideal is outstripping our ability to deliver. Too few first line doctors are available in many areas to provide primary care, at least 24-hour access and ingress. In the past few years in this country we have attempted to increase the number of physicians in training and to emphasize primary care. If we appropriately identify the needs and desires of the public we are serving, the New Health Practitioner may be seen to be a better solution than expensive and highly trained super-physicians. Also, importing foreign trained physicians robs other less developed countries—a policy not recommended to endear us to others. With our talents and resources, we should be able to solve our own problems and to aid others as we do it."*

Thirty-eight years later, the future then envisioned has become the norm in medicine. This book is therefore dedicated to the preceptors, nurses and medical corpsmen who pioneered a new health profession.

This book recounts the leadership of Dr. Eelkema in responding to two serious health care needs of the time: The shortage of primary health care workers and the so-called maldistribution of the health care services. It represents an important milestone in the history of medicine in North Dakota and in the U.S.

—DOUGLAS FENDERSON, Ph.D.

Former Director, Office of Special Programs
Bureau of Health Manpower Education, Washington, D.C.

Table of Contents

Introduction

Medicine in the Back of Beyond is the story of how a few people, with a passion for helping others, worked together and overcame powerful and deep-seated skepticism to extend the reach of health care into the remotest parts of our country.

In the late 1960s, the University of North Dakota was at the forefront of an effort to train "mid-level practitioners," a new kind of provider who could ease the physician's burden and bring health care where it is most needed. The effort was led by an innovative and progressive thinker, Dr. Robert Eelkema, with the critical support of then-President Tom Clifford.

Dr. Eelkema and his colleagues developed the novel MEDEX Program, the second in the nation to train and graduate independent-duty corpsmen who were returning from Vietnam with a wealth of skills, knowledge and experience in trauma medicine but no avenue to practice in the U.S. health care system.

This book describes the early and serendipitous opportunities that led to the birth of the MEDEX Program at UND and, later, how the UND Nurse Practitioner/Physician Assistant Program grew from it. Dr. Eelkema was in the right place at the right time to recognize and capture those opportunities for the ultimate benefit of an inestimable number of people.

Part autobiography, part history lesson, this books tells the stories of some of the program's graduates who went on to make an essential difference in the provision of health care services throughout the nation. Dr. Eelkema looks at his life, his roots, his values and family tragedy, and shares wisdom that comes only from introspection later in life.

Healing is a matter of time, but it is sometimes a matter of opportunity.

—HIPPOCRATES (460 BC–370 BC)

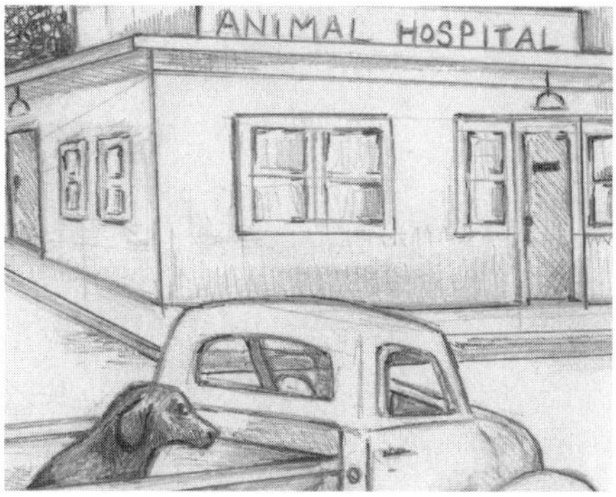

1

Digging into the Past

EMILY DICKINSON ONCE said "the past is not a package one can lay away." She was wrong, but only by one word. For years, decades in fact, I laid away a package called the past. Not a tidy package, but more like a dumpster that never made it to the dump. Had Emily added the word "forever" to the end of her thought, she would have captured the essence of the itch that chafed at my subconscious long enough that I finally reached the point where I could put off scratching it no longer.

About three years ago I finally mustered the nerve and energy to go out to the garage where I'd parked a small trailer years earlier in one of my self-delusional attempts to hold the past at bay. The trailer bulged with memories of my mother and father and their mothers and fathers and several generations back of parents, grandparents, great-grandparents, cousins and great-great- uncles who came from Holland and Germany and, ultimately, America.

One set of those grandparents produced seven children: one died in infancy, five were boys and one, a girl. That was my mother. All through their lives they saved *everything*. All the letters they ever got from any of their children. Personal effects such as furniture and photographs that, while treasured during their lives, became unwanted junk upon their deaths. None of my uncles wanted any of it, so they loaded all of it and dumped it off at my folks' house in Duluth, Minn.

Not that my parents knew what to do with it. Up into the attic went those memories and they sat undisturbed and collecting dust until after my parents died—my father in 1977 and my mother in 1980. When my brother, sister and I began breaking up the old household, nobody wanted any of the stuff up in the attic. Nobody meant I got it all. So I built a small white shed behind our home in Grand Forks, N.D., and put it all in there. There it stayed until the Great Flood of 1997, the one that produced news photos published around the world showing buildings engulfed in flames on streets waist-deep in the waters of the Red River of the North.

Reminiscent of the old song about the cat that kept coming back, the flood destroyed our home, but not the little white shed with *all that stuff*. I didn't know what to do with it so I packed it away and put it into one of those mini-storage lockers. I paid $33 a month for 10 years just so I wouldn't have to think about it. Finally, I got smart and bought a trailer. With the help of my son, Robbie, we shifted everything from mini-storage into the trailer and then moved the trailer into the garage. We closed the door and dusted our hands, satisfied at a job well done. The trailer, meanwhile, sat untouched for another few years until the day I pushed myself out there and started going through everything, piece by piece.

I found an awful lot of stories in there. I found my grandparents' wedding license and my grandfather's naturalization papers from the nineteenth century. There were hundreds of letters from my father, who owned a small typewriter and loved to write letters. Every time he wrote one, he put a carbon copy in and saved it in a filing cabinet.

My dad and mom were both born in Iowa. His mother, whose maiden name was Elizabeth Kaufman, was born in Schleswig-Holstein in 1850. She came over as a 12-year-old with her mother, who was widowed, and they settled in Chicago.

I have quite a record from my grandfather, Rienk Reinder Eelkema, who came over from Holland in 1860 when he was 20 (I think he got into a fight with his father). He was the eldest of six children, born in Oostmeer, Holland. He was a shoemaker by trade, so was his father, grandfather and great-grandfather before him. I've visited Oostmeer—it means East Lake, and in the town there was a lake with a river going through it. I've also visited his home in Iowa and it had a lake with a river running through it and they looked very much alike. I think people who came over from the "old country" tended to settle in areas that made them think of home. I'm sure of it.

By the way, there's an interesting story about the origin of the name, Eelkema. Before 1811, when Napoleon annexed Holland to his empire, the surname Eelkema did not exist. In fact, across Holland the use of surnames was not widespread at all. Napoleon ordered that everyone register a surname of their choice. People generally picked a name that suggested a favored quality like De Jongh, meaning young, or an occupation such as De Klerk or a geographical area such as De Vries, meaning someone from the province of Friesland. That's where my father's people were from. Strangely, even though Holland has no mountains at all, the name Van den Berg—meaning "of the mountain"—is popular. Perhaps it refers to the size of one's ego.

At any rate, before 1811, my great-great-grandfather's name was Eelkes. My grandmother was named simply Tadema. When they went to declare their surname they combined the two names to make Eelkema. Only three families in all of Holland registered that name. Basically they're all related to me.

Sometime after that, the men on my father's side began using the first name Rienk Reinder. That man's first son was named Reinders Rienk. Then, the first son would name his first son Rienk Reinder, and so on. When Ginny and I married in 1973, we'd each been through a divorce. I brought six kids to the marriage and she brought four. We then had one child together, a son, whom we named Cameron Rienk Reinder Eelkema. We called him Rienk.

Once you start digging into the past, it's hard to stop. Maybe it's the release of all that guilt built up for years doing what Emily Dickinson warned about. Anyway, around the same time as I was getting to know a lot more than I ever thought I wanted to know about my folks, my cousins and my uncles, I began poring over another long-forgotten archive.

As a young physician many years ago, one with a penchant for pushing the envelope of public health and rural medicine, I grandly told myself that if I ever accomplished something worthwhile I would write a book about it. It turns out that by the time I retired in 2000 from the School of Medicine at the University of North Dakota, something I initiated and guided over a period of 28 years had come together to revolutionize the delivery of health care in underserved areas.

In the early days of the 1970s, attention in the health care field was just beginning to focus on what were being called "New Health Practitioners." I learned quite a bit about that movement through a colleague named Dick Smith, whom I'd met at the University of Washington during my residency training in epidemiology.

Dick got a grant to start a nationwide program called MEDEX; the term was a contraction of French and Spanish words that mean 'extension of the doctor.' The MEDEX Program was aimed at areas of America—both urban and rural—where medical care was inaccessible or non-existent. The reason such areas were underserved by doctors was that too many had no desire or motivation to set up practice in areas outside their comfort zones, both cultural and financial. Dick wondered what might happen if the medical profession could somehow extend its reach into such areas without the need for full-time doctors.

His idea was to recruit medical corpsmen returning from combat duty in Vietnam and supplement their experience of treating combat injuries with the basics of non-injury medical care found in a typical clinic or emergency room. The result would be an individual who could serve more or less as the medical extension of a doctor. They would become physician assistants (PA) or nurse practitioners (NP). They wouldn't replace a doctor but could, with training and close mentoring from nearby physicians, treat and resolve many of the basic medical issues common to underserved communities.

As the founding chair of the Department of Community Medicine at University of North Dakota, I was immediately captivated by the idea. North Dakota has four, not-very-large municipal centers. Fargo, the biggest, has a population of about 130,000, which includes the city of West Fargo. After that, Bismarck has 61,000, Grand Forks 53,000 and Minot 40,000. Those are the places doctors tend to settle in North Dakota—if they decide to settle at all. We have always had a shortage of doctors, not just in the cities, but mostly in the hundreds of small towns throughout the state in rural areas, places many outsiders would consider to be in the middle of nowhere.

The very reason a medical school was founded in 1905 at the university in Grand Forks was to graduate doctors who would serve the rural medical needs of the state. Otherwise, there wouldn't be any doctors at all. Right about the time of Dick Smith's MEDEX initiative, North Dakota was embroiled in a political fight about the future of that medical school.

Until 1972, it had been a two-year medical school, offering basic science courses for first- and second-year students who then would go elsewhere to finish their medical degree. That's why I went off to the University of Washington. The problem was that once students earn the medical degree (M.D.) and complete residency, the overwhelming majority tend to settle into their careers within 100 miles of that area. North Dakota's two-year grads just weren't coming home to serve their home-state residents.

By agreeing to fund a conversion of the medical school to a full four years, the state legislature in 1973 extracted the promise that medical students—most of whom come from North Dakota—would be trained in primary care medicine so that when they graduated as doctors they would be ready to go to work in their home state.

The rural health problem was one of the reasons that maintaining a department of community medicine made sense. While being a country doc may sound like the ideal, easy life, the responsibility of providing everyday medical needs to people in not just one, but several surrounding small towns—people who have no other doctor to go to for miles—can be quite daunting. Those physicians who choose to serve in rural areas often love the freedom and independence, but at the same time they can become isolated from colleagues and pushed to the burnout stage. Eventually they are forced to leave the area for the ironically healthier lifestyle of a busy city physician.

I found out from Dick Smith that he was planning on starting MEDEX training programs in four regions of the country. I immediately set to work getting approval for the University of North Dakota to become one of those four sites. I was convinced that by extending the capabilities of a rural doctor's office through MEDEX training, we could make possible for doctors a much saner share of the burden, and simultaneously afford the citizens of the state greater access to needed care.

Within weeks of our initial efforts at organizing, we were in receipt in 1969 of a grant for $1.7 million from the Division of Health Manpower Research in the National Institutes of Health, out of Dr. Paul Sanazaro's office. It was the largest grant the university had ever received. Over the next 25 years, using scarcely a dollar of state or university money, we trained and graduated 1,100 PAs and NPs who deployed in underserved areas in North Dakota and, ultimately, into every one of the 49 other states in the Union

Thus, when I retired at age 70 in 2000, there was every reason for pride and satisfaction, knowing that those 1,100 graduates were helping tens of thousands of people who otherwise would have been shut out. Yet it was very difficult for me to feel anything at the time. The reason I retired had less to do with my age than with a personal tragedy that cloaked me in the blackest of depressions and stole away my zeal for doing anything at all.

Less than a year before, a senseless traffic accident only six days after his wedding, took the life of our beloved, youngest son, Rienk. He was the child Ginny and I had together, perfectly joining the two halves of our extended family in a most unlikely version of Yours, Mine and Ours. Rienk's 22 years to that point spanned almost the entire life of our medical extension program, infusing me countless times with the energizing joy and purpose necessary to keep our ambitious efforts humming. His uncanny ability to befriend everyone he came in contact with, to impart wisdom beyond his years, to make one glad to be alive, was irreplaceable.

After his death, I didn't think I could go on, so I put in my retirement papers. In my last year, my successor and friend, Dr. Jim Brosseau, took over the reins of the program. Meanwhile, I traveled across the country stopping in to see some of our graduates at work in their communities and to witness the difference they were making in the lives of the people they served. I took with me a tape-recorder and recorded about 35 different interview sessions. When I finished my travels I had the tapes transcribed with the intention of working them into a book about our program. But in all honesty, I was still stuck fast in grief and found it difficult to build an interest in anything.

Three things saved me. First was Ginny, whose devastation equaled my own. Together we grieved and sought solace in a variety of directions. Our own family of ten wonderful children and their children and all of their careers and love sustained us through the storm. Finally, there came a point in 2001 when I decided that if I was going to continue living I might as well go back to work.

It helped that I remembered the words of a colleague, a supremely skilled physician who had retired at 62. I would see him often during the years of his retirement—a very long and healthy retirement. He lived into his 90s and he once told me that as much as he enjoyed playing golf all the time, he wished he hadn't retired so early. His words were something to the effect of, "If I had known I was going to live this long I would have stayed a doctor."

That sentiment comes, I know, from a physician's life-long love for the practice of medicine. It was something I realized that I missed terribly. I got back in touch with a friend from medical school who operated a firm that hired doctors to work part-time shifts in rural emergency rooms in small cities in Minnesota and North Dakota. We talked and I told him that while I had more of a past than a future, I was interested in returning to medicine. So I became a physician again, charged once more with healing others, but mindful also of the ongoing responsibility to heal myself.

This year (2011), as I turned 81, I retired again. I still feel a great sadness and emptiness about Rienk, for it just seems so wrong for a parent to outlive a child. But Ginny and I have found some peace, and our friendship and love have gradually returned us to the ranks of the happy-to-be-alive.

All of which is a very long-winded way of getting back to the point that I haven't even made yet, and back to those old letters and clippings and transcripts that I have found myself sifting through in recent years. As I went from one archive to the other, from the roots of my family to the fruits of my labor, I began to see two story paths converging.

One is the story of who I am—although it certainly is no whoop-dee-do tale of the greatest thing since sliced bread. Who I am is really the story of Why I am. And to tell that story properly, to have any chance of arriving at an answer to that "why," I must start with the Rienk Reinders of my past. With the story of Uncle Louie and the Reverend Mister Grandpa Fred and my straight-laced, penny-pinching, fast ball-hurling father who thought he ran the show, and of my elegant, reserved mother who, in fact, did run the show but charitably, never let on, and off of whose sensitive block I am but a tiny chip.

The other story is the one that begins when a happy-go-lucky hayseed runs out of gas going uphill in a car that cost $89. He rolls backward downhill just long enough to appreciate that not everyone in this life was born with the gift for planting and raising a quarter-section of flax and potatoes and coming out of it with more money than he had going in.

I think we all reach a point in our lives where a turn in the road up ahead presents itself. It is up to each of us to have paid enough attention in the early and formative Rienk-Reinder years to know whether or not to take that turn. I am fortunate that the Who I became was able to recognize some of those turns in the road and took one now and then.

As I said, I once promised myself that if I ever accomplished something worthwhile, I'd write it out. For the longest time I felt that my success was all about creating better access to health care for those without, by training bright young men and women to provide that service as physician assistants and nurse practitioners. But I think now that what I really have accomplished, whether as a public health educator or a plain old country doc, was simply being able to recognize and help point out to others those fateful turns in the road up ahead.

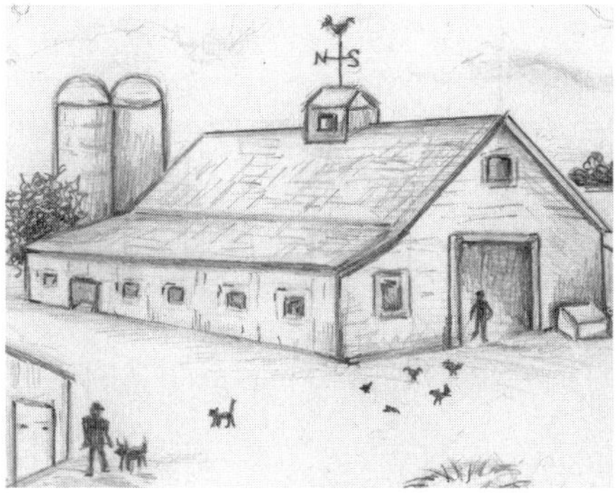

2

Extending the Reach

One summer in the late 1940s when I was about 16, I was working for my father with a crew doing combine harvesting for farmers all over the Midwest. We were in South Dakota one day when my friend Tom Wilson—everybody called him Screech—got his hand caught in a V-belt on a combine pickup. When he pulled his hand free, his little finger dangled at an impossible angle.

I rushed him into Plankington, the nearest town, where we knew there was a clinic. I followed Screech into that clinic where we found an old and very obese doctor sitting at a roll top desk. As soon as he saw Screech, he went into his lower right hand drawer and he brought out a pair of ancient and rusted scissors. He took Screech's hand and said, "Son, you're not gonna need that finger." And he cut it off right there; bandaged him up, and we went back to work.

Another guy in our crew had a bad sore throat and he went into a doctor's office in the nearest small town. The doctor examined his throat and said, "Son, you don't need those tonsils."

He took him into a back room and took out the tonsils. Well, he bled for a long time. He lost nearly 15 pounds before he got better. Later, in medical school, I would learn that taking out infected tonsils is not what you call great medical care.

Then there was the day when I was out cultivating near the small town of Grafton, N.D., and developed a terrible toothache. I went into Grafton and saw a dentist who said, "You've got an infected wisdom tooth and that should come out." So he lightly anesthetized me. He had a pliers, a chisel and a hammer and he used them all. He dug and he yanked and he pulled and he finally got that wisdom tooth out. I asked him how much and he said, "Well, would $20 be okay?" So I gave him a $20 bill but I didn't go back to get the other three wisdom teeth taken out. That was enough for me.

Medicine in rural places is always a problem, and not just for the patient. During the nearly ten years that I spent working in rural emergency rooms—in towns big enough to afford one—I experienced my share of difficult moments when I felt alone and unsupported in the midst of a medical crisis. That is not uncommon out in the countryside. When there's an ice storm and you get an automobile accident with multiple injuries, you're the only one to take care of them. You don't have a helicopter or an ambulance to send them to a city hospital for specialist care. You're the specialist and sometimes it can get a little bit exciting.

One night we had an older man brought in who had been found unconscious in his home. We worked very hard under the great pressure of time and finally revived him. Later, when I came into the room to see how he was doing, he said angrily, "I don't know why you tried to save me. My wife died. I don't want to live. Why did you do that to me?"

Simple depression—or even serious depression—is one thing to deal with, but a big frustration of working in small communities late at night is having a patient come in who is having a psychotic break, or someone who is suicidal or manic. There is a severe need in rural communities for inpatient psychiatric care, but the vast majority of small hospitals have no room for mental health or psychiatric care—or chemical dependency for that matter.

If it happens in the middle of the night you call up places within 50 or 100 miles and you might find a doctor on call. Usually he's unaware if there's an appropriate bed available or not. Sometimes you can tell they're not really interested in accepting a patient. Often they are difficult to talk to because their English is not very good. Most of the time they say I's impossible. I found that the only time I really could get a patient admitted somewhere is if I said this patient is suicidal and needs to be on a suicide watch. That might not necessarily be true, but it does mean I can an get that patient into a sheltered environment. Your job in that situation is to protect the patient and the public.

Most mental hospitals are run by government agencies, usually by the state. Most are underfunded, and don't have adequate medical staff. And most don't have serious or acute beds available. That's something that gets very little attention. You're really left to the lions. It's no wonder that in so many rural areas, physicians are hard to come by.

The state of North Dakota used to offer loans to its two-year medical students. If they came back to practice in a rural area after earning their medical degree, the state would forgive one-fifth of the loan every year. Sounded like a good idea, but the bad part came when doctors who took those loans came back and started to look on themselves as indentured servants. As soon as the loan was paid off they were off and running. It just seems like common sense that you can't own a person and make them feel good. Even so, it was a point we didn't fully appreciate when we started our MEDEX Program.

Our involvement in MEDEX was something of a fluke. Shortly after I'd finished my public health/epidemiology residency and returned to UND in 1968, I attended a convention in Philadelphia of the American Public Health Association. There I ran into my friend, Dick Smith, whom I'd first met at the University of Washington. We were each headed to a different session that day in the Bellevue Stratford hotel (also known as the hotel where Legionnaire's Disease originated) and didn't have much time to catch each other up on our careers. I knew Dick had just returned from a stint in the Peace Corps and as I walked him to a bank of elevators I asked what he was working on now. He said, "MEDEX." The elevator arrived then and as he was getting on I said, "What the hell is MEDEX?" He quickly handed me a card and told me to give him a call.

When I called a few days later he explained the idea of taking independent-duty corpsmen from Vietnam and reintroducing them to civilian practice in rural communities. I said, "Boy, that's something we need in North Dakota." A lot of our rural doctors were approaching retirement without anyone lined up to replace them. In fact, many of them kept putting off their retirement because of the desperate need for their services.

Dick told me that if I could get the state medical association and the medical school to approve our involvement, we were in. He already had lined up Dartmouth College, the University of Utah and the Charles R. Drew medical school in Los Angeles. We would be the representative of the Midwest under the MEDEX demonstration grant.

I was almost certain I could get the backing of the UND School of Medicine. The dean at the time, Dr. Ted Harwood, had been in charge while I was a student and was the man who'd hired me to start the Department of Community Medicine.

The first thing I did when I got off the phone with Dick was to look up the Board of Councilors for the North Dakota Medical Association. There were nine councilors, each representing a specific geographical region in the state. I immediately boiled it down to the bottom line: I only needed to win the support of five of them.

To start my lobbying for that support, I convened a large meeting at the Pow Wow room of the Westward Ho, a venerable old motel in Grand Forks. We had lots of booze flowing and I was able to win over a couple of councilors right away. It turned out that most of those in favor of MEDEX represented the rural regions. They knew firsthand what the needs were. Those against it were the doctors in the Bismarck and Fargo areas. They saw MEDEX as a threat to their professionalism and worried that these former corpsmen would be totally unqualified to do what we thought we could train them to do.

Perhaps because North Dakota has more rural than urban areas, the medical association approved our involvement by a 5-4 vote. Interestingly, once the program got going and began proving its worth, some of the doctors who pleaded with the association not to support it, ended up as our advocates.

By that point I'd recruited Judy DeMers from the UND College of Nursing to help get the MEDEX Program running. Judy had been teaching a valuable clinical course to second-year medical students and also to senior-year nurses. She and I went to Seattle to meet with Dick Smith, and there we wrote our application for a grant from the Division of Health Manpower Research in the National Institutes of Health. I hand-carried it to the NIH offices in Bethesda, Md.—something I made a point of doing from then on with every grant application we made.

In Bethesda, I met with Dr. Paul Sanazaro, who headed the department and his assistant, Doug Fenderson. It turned out Fenderson was from the small town of Streeter, N.D. His dad had been the telegrapher there. Needless to say, his immediate support played a very important role. In that meeting, I found out that Sanazaro's office wanted to fund programs that were heavy on research and less so on practical application. I wanted no part of a research-oriented program. I wanted hands-on medical people in the communities delivering health care. Sanazaro and Fenderson were so taken with our plans that they set up a special review for our project. Within three weeks they gave us about $1,700,000. With it we were able to recruit not only independent-duty corpsmen, but preceptors—doctors in the field who would mentor and supervise our graduates.

It wasn't long before we hit our first speed bump. We had the money but we didn't have a specific plan for what we were going to teach these corpsmen. To that end, Dick Smith had circulated questionnaires among the chairs of various medical school departments across the country. He asked them, essentially, what our students would need to know to function as physician assistants in a rural area.

The trouble is, those department heads were academically oriented and very urban. They had never gone out to a rural area to understand the unique medical needs of that population. They were ultimately afraid to go with something other than their snug harbor and university setting. As their questionnaires came back, Smith tallied the requirements they listed. To work them all into a curriculum would have required a student to spend 14 years and 10 months of study. In other words, our students would have to go through everything those chairmen had gone through plus more.

We needed to get it down to 18 months. Dick and his assistants then decided on a different tack—a task analysis and a needs assessment. They selected about 150 procedures common to family practice medicine and sent new questionnaires to a large group of family practice doctors. For each procedure listed, they asked doctors to make one of three choices: Would you delegate this to an assistant? Would you never delegate it? Would you sometimes delegate it?

From those answers, Smith and his assistants designed a curriculum that focused on the realistic needs of a practitioner in a rural area. One of key considerations was that the group we hoped to train already had invaluable experience. They were bright people, most of whom had gone through two years of intense medical training at the Army's Fort Sam Houston. They had spent at least a year in combat as independent-duty corpsmen in outfits such as the Green Berets, Delta Force and other special-forces units. They were steeped in trauma, so what they really had to learn was the more practical, everyday routine of a typical family practice doc.

It wasn't long before we developed our curriculum into a flexible, modular program. It began with a four-week introductory training session followed by three to four months in the field working alongside a physician-preceptor. The students then came back to campus for a didactic segment, concentrating on common medical situations that included emergency medicine, acute care, and some surgery. Then they went out again and practiced what they'd learned, overseen by their preceptor. They would return to campus once more for a several-week didactic session that emphasized chronic conditions. Then they went back to their preceptors and tried to put it all together.

We had developed a list of physicians willing to serve as preceptors. They were all North Dakota doctors and not faculty members of the medical school. We paid them an honorarium and most were pleased to be involved.

However, the initial method we used to pair each student with a preceptor was flawed. We had a system whereby three preceptors would interview three likely students and then select the one they wanted to work with. The problem was that the students had no say in the process. By matching them like that there was a lot of room for error and for attrition. We later realized that it would be much better to have a potential student and a physician already living and working in their community to seek each other out and, essentially, select themselves.

For a time, we were a bastard program at UND that really didn't have a home on campus. We held our initial lectures anywhere we could find room. At the very beginning we used the Methodist church in Grand Forks. Once or twice we had to go to Minot and use the facilities at Minot State University's School of Nursing.

I was able to recruit two highly qualified nurses from that school to assist. I had actually worked closely with both Judy DeMers and Mickey Knutson since 1964, when I started the Department of Community Medicine. At the time, the UND medical school was still a two-year school. Medical students were taught the basic science course and didn't begin hands-on medicine until their third year. With input from Mickey and Judy, we devised a special course for senior nursing students and sophomore medical students in public health epidemiology.

We recruited patients from the local Alcoholics Anonymous, the developmental disabilities group, the local rehab center, and those discharged from the local hospital with chronic problems. We assigned patients to a team that included medical and nursing students. It was the first exposure those medical students had with live patients. We taught them how to interview patients in detail, one of the most useful skills a physician can develop.

Judy and Mickey eventually transferred to the Department of Community Medicine full time where they became absolutely indispensable to the MEDEX Program. Both acted as counselors. They were excellent listeners and very experienced nurses with all the necessary qualities of insight, wisdom and understanding. One of the things they did was to share the duties with me of visiting the preceptor sites where our students were training in the field. We checked the sites quite often to make sure the student and doctor were working well together. Often we'd use airplanes from the UND Center for Aerospace Sciences to make four or five visits a day around the state. (By doing that we were also giving student pilots an opportunity to build their flight hours.)

We graduated our first class in January 1972, the third university in the country—after Dick Smith's program in Seattle and one at Duke University—to send a MEDEX class into the field. But just because they graduated didn't mean they were accepted by the medical community or even by their potential patients. There was a long adjustment period during which our graduates ran into doctors, nurses and administrators who wouldn't cooperate with them and refused to recognize their competency, even though each was accredited by both the American Nurses Association and the American Physician Assistants Association, an arm of the American Medical Association.

Many states outlined very specific procedures as to what these graduates could and could not do in terms of practicing medicine. Others left it up to the doctor with whom they were practicing—but added some notable exceptions, like delivering babies and doing surgery.

Some states were more lenient than others, and depending on the liberality of the state they would recognize either the PA or the NP accreditation. Some even recognized both, but then there was Ohio, where laws at the time were so rigid and restrictive it was hard for students to stay there. Prescription privileges became a *bette noir*, but pretty soon most states were allowing PAs and NPs to write prescription for antibiotics. Some were even allowing narcotics, with a countersignature from a physician.

It got to the point where much of my time was spent meeting with state boards of medicine and nursing to sort out the various legalities and permissions. Even with the early instances of feet-dragging by some states and physician organizations, positive reports from doctors in the field about the efficacy of using trained personnel to extend their reach began to tell. Where initially there was an awful lot of supervision and closeness demanded by state regulating authorities, after a while that became more relaxed. People were finding out that our PAs and NPs could actually help them.

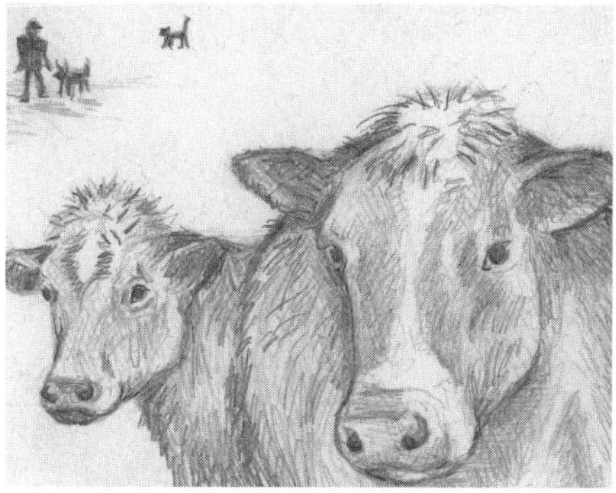

3

Evil Stuff in Iowa

WHILE I WAS a veterinary student at the University of Minnesota in Minneapolis in the 1950s, I decided one day to donate blood at the local hospital. By coincidence, I met a nurse who had worked in a hospital in Mankato, Minn., about 80 miles southwest of Minneapolis, during the time I was born there in 1930. The nurse told me that more than half the children born in the weeks just before and after my birth had died of diarrheal dehydration.

Years later, when I applied for a passport, I ran into delays because my birth certificate identified me only as "Baby Boy Eelkema." I had to get an affidavit from my folks saying that Baby Boy Eelkema and Robert Cameron Eelkema were one and the same person. It was also my chance to ask them why my actual name wasn't on the birth certificate in the first place. It turned out that my mother and father were very aware of the diarrheal dehydration at the time. In fact, they didn't think I was going to live, so they didn't name me until I got out of the hospital.

For my mother, this wasn't just a silly precaution. Nine years before I was born, she gave birth to her first child, a daughter, whom she named Barbara. But she lived only three days. In those days there was still a very high mortality rate among infants. We would hear stories as children of distant relatives from the nineteenth century who had lost children at tender ages.

I would later learn that in the middle of the nineteenth century, a family would need to have nine children, on average, just to have three of them live to adulthood. In any event, the death of my sister, Barbara, sent my mother into a long depression which didn't really lift until 1927, when my brother, Herman Harrison Eelkema, was born.

I grew up in the 1930s when childhood diseases like measles, mumps, whooping cough, rubella and diphtheria were considered very dangerous and very contagious. If one child in the family came down with an infectious disease, the Public Health people would come along and put a placard on your front door stating that this house is quarantined for two weeks. There were times when my sister, Ruth, would come down with mumps or measles, which meant my brother and I were quarantined for two weeks. Then he'd get it and my sister and I were quarantined. Then I'd get it and they were both quarantined. I'd be out of school sometimes for six weeks. Compounded with chicken pox, you ended up missing a lot of school.

We were fortunate that both my mother and father were teachers. We continued our learning even though we were out of school. Nowadays, with childhood immunizations having essentially wiped out those old childhood diseases, the only time kids miss school is when they have a little fever or a cold and then usually only one or two days.

When I was 16 or 17 I developed a particularly virulent and mysterious illness. Our doctor made a house call and gave me something for my fever but my mother got panicky and invited a Christian Science reader to come in. Finally she went to an ear, nose and throat specialist and he put me in the hospital. I was in an open alcove and spitting up and having a hard time breathing. They brought in a young man with similar symptoms and put him in the bed beside me in the open alcove. A couple of nights later, he died. Finally they took a swab of my throat. By the time I was getting better they diagnosed diphtheria. After that they put me in an isolation ward without any bathroom. I was laid up for quite some time. But I did get better.

Diphtheria was a very serious disease with a 12 to 20 percent fatality rate. Later on, in my epidemiology training, I saw a case of diphtheria in a nursing mother who later died. A very sad affair, particularly since diphtheria, by then, was a preventable disease. All you had to do was get a DPT (diphtheria, pertussis and tetanus) immunization. We found in our studies that 15 to 20 percent of the population at the time was just not availing themselves of vaccines and were still vulnerable to childhood diseases. Each generation forgets about doing it. And since too many people don't understand the seriousness of childhood diseases, every once in a while these diseases will pop up again, which is unfortunate.

The success of vaccinations in eliminating childhood disease is a human achievement too often taken for granted. The story of the eradication of small pox alone is such a beautiful story. That we have eliminated it from our lexicon is absolutely amazing. (By the way, a medical school classmate of mine, William Foege, told the story of how small pox was eliminated and eradicated in India in a wonderful book called "House on Fire.")

During my residency in epidemiology I learned that most of the contagious part of childhood diseases occurs two weeks before a child comes down with symptoms. So the quarantining of cases back then didn't really do any good. Once you started showing the symptoms, the contagiousness of the disease was almost nil. It was the people whose symptoms hadn't yet shown, but who were walking around incubating the disease, who were the most contagious. We just were not aware then. We didn't know about how it worked.

Given my experiences, I suppose it's not surprising that while in medical school I became extremely interested in infectious diseases. I read Paul de Kruif's wonderful book, "Microbe Hunters," and the subject became kind of an obsession with me. I thought then that it was probably the direction I wanted to go in life. I just didn't know how I was going to get there.

Actually, there were many times in my life when I wondered how I would get from point A to point B. My personality is such that I never did a lot of worrying about it. I more or less did my wondering and then started taking small, sometimes bumbling steps forward, and things happened. Forward movement will almost always lead to a solution to a problem. I attribute that knowledge to my mother and father. They were forced by circumstance to keep their wits about them so they could make a life for their family. Both were not just forward movers, they were forward thinkers. The fact that each of them was also stricken by the awful influenza pandemic of 1918 that took between 50 and 100 million lives worldwide—and then raised a doctor son who fell in love with public health medicine—is certainly curious. Undoubtedly, it helped shape my ability to keep stepping to the front.

Both my mother and father were born in Iowa, a state of hearty and self-sufficient farm people, like so much of the Midwest. My father was the eleventh of twelve children. He lost two of his brothers in their 20s to tuberculosis. As a young man he developed what is called a Ghon complex—a walled off granuloma of TB—but his immune system was able to fight it off. He'd made plans to become a plumber but when he applied for an apprenticeship, no one in the plumbing business would touch him with a ten-foot pole because of that TB connection.

He was only 16 when his mother and father died in 1909. Uncertain of what to do, he took one of the many immigrant trains set up by the railroads to promote settlement of the wide open spaces of the West. It's the way little towns in rural states like North Dakota attracted thousands of settlers who stepped off of those trains at some unsettled backwater area and instantly created a community of people with like-minded religious and cultural backgrounds.

Immigrants were charged lower than normal fares on those trains, but they had to ride in the older rail cars which usually were crowded with people carrying all of their worldly possessions. That included pigs, chickens, cows and even a horse or two. My father paid for his fare out west by caring for the animals in those cars all the way out to Quincy, Wash. When he got out there, however, he became so lonely he wanted to go home right away. He went to a pharmacist in Quincy, a complete stranger, and told him his sad story. The man took pity on him and loaned him enough money to take an empty immigrant train back to Iowa.

I wasn't aware of that chapter of his life until 1939 when we all drove out west in my father's new Studebaker. We visited relatives in San Francisco but we also drove up to Quincy, and stopped at that same pharmacy. The pharmacist, now very old, still remembered my dad from 30 years earlier. It was quite a touching and poignant moment when Dad proudly repaid the man his loan—quite a lesson for a nine-year-old as well.

At any rate, instead of becoming a plumber, my father had become a college man. He'd enrolled at Upper Iowa University in Fayette, Iowa in 1911. Nobody else in my father's family ever made it to college and even he might not have made it if not for his skill at baseball. Living then in Tripoli, Iowa (pronounced *TRIP*-o-la), he played short stop and second base and once in a while he'd pitch for the town baseball team. The baseball coach of the team in Fayette, which was not too far from Tripoli, recruited Dad to come to school at Upper Iowa and play—probably among the very first sports scholarships ever given out. Anyway, at Upper Iowa he became captain of both the baseball and basketball teams.

In that same year, a young woman named Ruth Naomi Young arrived in Fayette and enrolled at Upper Iowa. Her path eventually crossed that of Herman Eelkema and they fell in love. There was one slight problem, however: her father didn't like her boyfriend.

Born in Chelsea, Iowa, Ruth was the daughter of Emma Kiefer, whose mother had emigrated from Bavaria, Germany in the mid-nineteenth century, and Frederick Young whose father was a London bookseller who moved his trade to Brooklyn and eventually Iowa.

The bookseller eventually became something of a well-off

gentleman-farmer. When he died, the land went to his two boys—my future grandfather, Fred, and great-uncle, John. Neither was a good businessmen nor a good farmer and it wasn't long before they lost everything. Fred got religion, became a born-again Christian and, soon, a Methodist minister.

I can say from personal experience, he was a very strict, Bible-pounding minister. When I was about five years old we lived fairly close to Grandpa Fred and Grandma Emma, and in the summer I'd be farmed out there for a few weeks. On Sundays we went to church to hear him preach and afterwards we'd drive around in his 1932 Plymouth. Eventually we'd park in the middle of some small town. I'd stay in the car with grandma playing cards. I'd ask where Grandpa went and she'd say, "Oh, he's out trying to save someone."

He was actually going into bars in those small towns to see if he couldn't get people to quit drinking. He was a member of the Women's Christian Temperance Union, and I well remember when he had me sign a pledge not to drink intoxicating beverages. Every time I have a beer or a glass of wine I remember it. He was well-meaning, but he was also fairly profane. Because he didn't make much money preaching, he had to milk cows and work farms in his spare time. And you could hear from a long ways off swearing at the cows whenever they gave him trouble.

At night Grandma Emma gave us cocoa and crackers. Grandpa Fred liked to play solitaire. He'd clear the table and then take off the oilcloth and lay out his cards. But if someone from the parish came to the door, he'd throw the oilcloth back on the table over the cards. I said to him once, "Why are you doing that, Grandpa?" He said, "Well, some of my parishioners don't like me to play cards."

Even at the age of five, I recognized the duplicity of that.

Grandpa Fred served as pastor in small towns all across Iowa. Every two years he'd put all of the family's belongings on a railroad car and ship them off to a new church in a new town. He moved to Fayette specifically so his children could attend Upper Iowa.

After meeting and falling in love, my future mother and father graduated from Upper Iowa in 1916. They planned to marry and work as teachers or school administrators. But Fred refused to give his blessing. It may have had something to do with the way my father worked his way through college. Like many of his fellow immigrants from Holland, my father was a conservative man and very careful with his money. On the other hand, I think there was a bit of the renegade Dutchman in him. Because he owned, at various times during his college days, a pool hall, a bowling alley and a barbershop—pretty evil stuff in Iowa.

So after they graduated, Dad applied to the school district in Drayton, N.D., for a job as the school superintendent. I found his letter of application in the trailer. In it he told them that he'd taught in a one-room schoolhouse, played baseball and basketball and had majored in administration. Again, it was the baseball that worked the charm. They hired him as the superintendent at the age of 23. When he got to Drayton, he was immediately recruited to the town team where he earned $75 a game. The school board, meanwhile, paid him $450 as year for being the superintendent.

My mother, in the meantime, got a job as superintendent of schools in Troy, Iowa. They may have gone their separate ways, but there were an awful lot of love letters going back and forth between Troy and Drayton. In September 1917, my dad went back to Iowa, and he and my mother eloped. Grandpa Fred never knew about it. The only reason I know about it was because of the old letters and my mother's wedding diary stuffed into the attic/white house/storage unit/trailer/garage.

But that wasn't the end of it. Grandpa Fred still had some cards hidden beneath the oilcloth.

After my folks' elopement, my mother moved up to Drayton and became a teacher; she taught English, math and agriculture. She said she knew absolutely nothing about agriculture but she was always one page ahead of the class in the textbook. In going through all of the stuff in the trailer, I found that she was well-liked as a teacher and won several awards for teaching.

When the First World War came along, my dad joined the army and they sent him to telegraphers school. He was assigned to

Fort Taylor in Kentucky where he went through officer candidate school and became a second lieutenant. My mother, meanwhile, moved back to Iowa to live with her parents.

On the train to Fort Taylor, Dad got to exchanging life stories about growing up in Iowa with the older man sitting next to him. A lot of the things they each mentioned sounded very similar. Finally, the other man said, "Well, what's your name?" And Dad said, "Well, it's a kind of unusual. You'll never remember it." The guy says, "Try me." So Dad said, "My name is Eelkema." The man next to him said, "That's my name." And he turned out to be my father's older brother, Louie.

He was 25 years older than Dad and had moved away after my dad was born. They'd never seen each other and obviously didn't know each other. After that, though, they became very good friends and visited each other quite often. Louie was the barber at the Palace Hotel in San Francisco. I remember going out there as a kid—on that trip where we stopped in Quincy, Wash. I got my hair cut by him in a barbershop with 24 chairs. Those were the days when people came in and got a shave as well as a haircut. I'd never seen a barbershop that big.

Anyway, Dad became a second lieutenant and was proud as peaches. He was transferred to Fort Sill, Okla., and on the way there, his train stopped in Tama, Iowa where he got off to see my mother. She was just recovering from the flu of 1918. My father announced that he was going to Fort Sill and Ruth was going with him. But my grandfather, Fred, said, "No, you're not. Not without being married."

So he went down and got a marriage license at the Tama courthouse and he married them on the spot. Not a word was mentioned about the small fact that they had already been married for year. A few hours later, Dad got on the train again to Fort Sill.

My mother joined him later, when she'd recovered from the flu. In her wedding diary she said that when she was going through Des Moines she could see the stacks of pine boxes for the doughboys who had died of the flu. She met my father in Kansas City and they had a two-day honeymoon and went back to Fort Sill.

About the second or third day they were down there, Dad came down with a fever and the chills. My mother insisted he go to the dispensary. He did and was immediately hospitalized. She was able to visit him but only for a short while. He was more or less quarantined. My mom tells about the five young soldiers who came through at various times and had the bed next to my dad. Each one of them died of the flu. Later, Dad described looking out the window and seeing the pine boxes piled high.

But he survived, and that November the war ended. He got out of the service without ever having to go to Europe. I have his uniform and cavalry boots. I sent it in for cleaning and they took off all the buttons and I've got 'em all, but I don't know where they go.

Incidentally, my father never forgot how to cut hair and he cut mine and my brother's hair up to the time he died in 1977, just short of his 85th birthday.

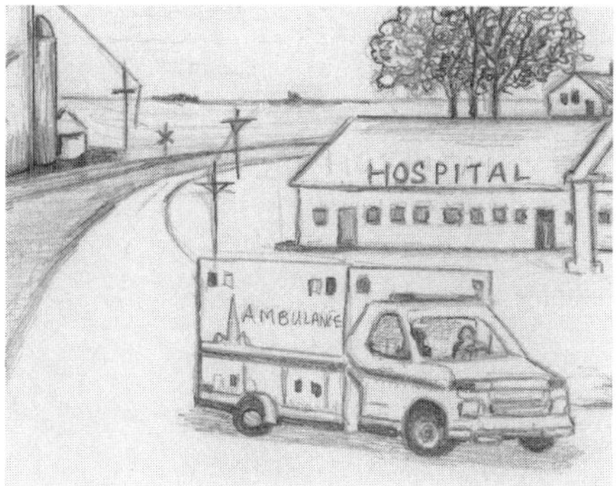

4

One of the Good Guys

DECEMBER 18, 2001

I AM IN Vinton, Iowa, the home of Harold Vanscoy whom I have just interviewed. Harold is a graduate of our very first MEDEX Program in 1972. He is also a long-time friend. A graduate of the University of North Dakota, he served three tours of duty in Vietnam, from 1967 to 1969 with the Third Special Forces Group. In 1969 he was assigned to the special operations outfit known as Delta Force. After the war, following his graduation from our program, he worked as a physician assistant in the UND Student Health Service for about 17 years. He has been a PA in the clinic in Vinton ever since.

Harold is a slight man. I think he must be an inch or two shorter than I am, and I am about 5'10". He probably weighs 140 or 150 pounds. He never had much of a pot on him. He must have a way of controlling his diet. He certainly is a heck of a lot smaller than I am but he has always been that way. He has a mustache and is a good-looking guy. He comports himself well. The clinic people like him and he tends to get along well with people and is just a nice fellow. He was exactly the kind of student we wanted for that first MEDEX class.

His 91-year-old mother died in 2000 and he couldn't be at my retirement dinner where he was slated to be one of the speakers. Harold's father died quite early in his childhood so he was mostly raised by his mother.

During our talk I learned that in his Special Forces training, Harold had to choose a specialty area, such as communications, engineering, demolition, intelligence. Harold chose medicine.

"They couldn't afford to send physicians out doing that kind of work so they wanted someone trained more than the average military guy was trained," he told me. "So they had this real extensive school. They put you through basic sciences and they put you through just about everything, along with your other Special Forces training. After that, you had to cross-train with all the other specialties in weapons and demolitions and so forth."

In Vietnam, whenever he was not on a combat operation, Harold conducted medical clinics in field camps and trained local mercenaries to be medics. Once he left camp, his role reverted to that of a combat soldier and he would lead those mercenaries into combat.

During his three years in Vietnam, Harold was awarded several medals, including a Silver Star for heroism. He was also wounded three times: once in the face from shrapnel, once in the butt, and the third time, the most serious, in the abdomen. He recalled that one in particular.

"I was laid out in the field for about two days before they came and got me, so I was pretty sick," he said. "I had a colon that was perforated. When I got off the helicopter, I was really sick to my stomach but I saw this pretty little blonde face. And then I got taken into surgery and when I woke up, she is the nurse standing there by my bed. Her name was Carol.

"It was kind of funny but every day I started feeling a little bit better, so we started sneaking outside. She worked the day shift. She would go home and clean up and then come back and visit me. So we started taking walks together. We went down to the beer place and had a few beers once in a while. We kind of had this little romance going so I kind of drug my feet leaving Vietnam. I was supposed to leave a week after they operated on me but I hung around for about three weeks. Then, after I got back home, I wrote her a few letters and after that I just never heard from her again."

While he was recuperating in Vietnam, Harold had a visit from Colonel Harold Rowe, the commander of all Special Forces in Southeast Asia. He had signed his papers to re-enlist, but the colonel told him, "Why don't you go back home to Denver and do something else? You have paid your dues."

So he mustered out of the Army and went home. But the dramatic change from war to a civilian lifestyle confused him.

"I got a little depressed and I didn't know what I wanted to do for sure," he said. "In the meantime, all those guys that I went to college or high school with, they would all call me up and say, 'Well, let's go out to lunch' and then I would end up drinking with them and things just weren't working out. I think, in retrospect, I was about half clinically depressed. I think I probably lost a part of me when I got out of Special Forces and I didn't recognize it at that time.

"My brother and I walked into a bar one night. He plays $5 worth of that Barry Sadler "Green Beret" song on the jukebox and it started two or three fights. And I thought to myself, 'I have to get out of Denver.'

"Then this buddy of mine, an internist in Vermont whom I'd met in the Army, told me about this MEDEX program they were starting at Dartmouth College in New Hampshire. I flew out to Vermont and we went over to Dartmouth and visited their MEDEX people. They said, 'Why don't you apply?' I told them I'd think about it. They also told me that North Dakota was starting a MEDEX program. So I sent an application to North Dakota and they invited me out for an interview."

Finding that the MEDEX program seemed a perfect fit for what he wanted, Harold remembers being conflicted.

"I was kind of teetering whether I was going to go to MEDEX school or back into Special Forces. I even went as far as flying back to North Carolina and I talked to all the big shots in Special Forces and they said, yeah, they would welcome me back with open arms. You know, I went through that Special Forces school which was extremely difficult. There were 67 of us that started the class and only 11 of us graduated. And as I gained experience it just became part of me. And I think maybe my personality liked that kind of work and I enjoyed the medical part of it and I liked to help people and I also liked the combat part of it. I have always liked trauma medicine. I have been exposed to a lot of it and I suffered a lot of it and, I don't know, I was good at it. I just kind of had a natural knack. I just kind of had a sixth sense about things.

"In the meantime, North Dakota invited me out for an interview and I thought, well, I will interview up there before I make a decision. By the time I got back to Denver from the interview they had accepted me and I just had to make a decision. So I went to North Dakota, basically because it was the first one that started. Dartmouth had accepted me too but I think it was six more months before it started."

As I mentioned, those early graduates often faced a tough time breaking into the fairly hidebound world of medicine with their brand-new certifications. During his MEDEX training, and even afterward, Harold faced some of those hurdles. While he'd been trained to take the burden of care off the shoulders of a doctor, many of those physicians were slow to cooperate. The PA position was so new, they didn't trust it and felt threatened.

"The PA profession was basically designed to help physicians and be aligned with the medical profession," Harold said. "I think that taught me to work with physicians rather than against them. Except for a couple of physicians, most of the Grand Forks community accepted us pretty quickly.

"I think we had two or three doctors who were basically against us doing anything. I tried to develop a rapport with them. One day I started getting in this doctor's face and I said, 'You know, why don't you teach me this?' He got happy because I asked him to teach me. He was like the orthopedic surgeons. I would say, 'Geez, Dr. so and so, why don't you tell me about this or this or this or help me do this.' I developed a rapport with most of the physicians pretty rapidly. I think the North Dakota program gave us the flexibility to do that. I don't think you would have had that ability to learn as much as we did."

Interestingly, some of those doctors who opposed the program became its staunchest supporters over time. Harold told me about the time Dr. Lloyd Ralston, who was then chairman of the State Board of Medical Examiners, asked him to testify at a meeting about the PA profession.

"A couple of the doctors on the board didn't want the PAs to do anything at all. So I went down there (to the state capitol in Bismarck) and I think it was Dr. Phil Dahl who just chewed my ass and said, 'You guys have no right to do this and no right to do that,' blah, blah, blah, blah. So I just sat very calmly and told them that, you know, this is our education and this is what we can do and I think our profession is geared to working with physicians. We are not combative; we are here to help and not disrupt. Well, after the meeting, he kind of calmed down, and we talked for a few minutes and he wanted to go have a beer. So we went and had a beer and he was fine after that."

Harold is right. Phil Dahl became one of the program's foremost supporters.

Harold told me another story that was almost exactly the opposite—a very young doctor who cooperated almost to a fault. This happened in Grand Forks, when Harold was with the UND Student Health Service.

"I had an emergency surgery one day. A guy got into a fight in a bar and he got a knife right in the spleen. He was bleeding out. I was on call so I called Dr. Harold Tarpley's house and Ginny answered the phone and I said, 'I need Tarp at Deaconess right now.' Ginny says, 'Well, I can't disturb him, he is down stairs meditating." I said, 'Ginny, I need him right now.' So Tarp finally comes to the phone and I said, 'Tarp, I need you at Deaconess right now' and I didn't tell him why or nothing and he hung up on me.

"So I am thinking, 'Oh shit, what am I going to down now?' Less than five minutes later, Dr. Tarpley comes busting through those swinging doors and all he had on was his bikini underwear. He ran all the way from his home in his underwear. He says, 'What's wrong?' And I said, 'This guy is going to surgery. Dr. Dailey is in there already, getting him to sleep.' I wish I had had a camera that night; he had his bald head and his hair sticking up and his bikini underwear. Anyway, we get the guy into surgery and Tarp saved the guy's life.

"Later, there was the night Dr. Dailey was working hard in the emergency room and there were some people in there who were kind of what you'd call not nice people. He came walking by and he put his arm around me and he said, 'Harold, remember one thing in this business. A lot of these people are not going to pay you for what you do. I have it figured out it is between 10 and 15 per cent. And, you know what? That is OK. Accept it. That is your community service.' He was right. Times have changed now, a lot of guys don't think that way anymore."

I asked Harold what he remembered of his days in the Student Health Service. "There's a bunch of cases from those days that stick in your brain," he said. "There were some things that you do over the years that are really special. I remember this gal came in, kind of nondescript. She just looked terrible. High fever. Abdominal pain, pelvic pain, etc. She had a white count of 30-some thousand. So I called (Dr.) Jim Brosseau and told him this gal needs to be in the hospital, she is sicker than hell. He took her over there and he called me back a little while later. She had toxic shock syndrome. It was the first case ever in North Dakota."

From my own recollection of those days when Harold was in Grand Forks, I remember the feeling of pride that swelled up every time I saw him in action. We gave him a new identity, as a physician assistant and he gave the university top notch care. Those students he saw had no idea how lucky they were.

"There was a guy at the university," he told me. "He came in one day with just some shortness of breath and a cough. He saw somebody else the first time he was in and he came in again and saw somebody else. Anyway they sent him over to the Grand Forks Clinic but the guy kept getting worse. And he kept getting bounced around. He finally came into my office, gasping for breath. He had dilated veins on his chest. It turns out he had a big tumor in his media-sternum. He had superior vena cava syndrome. And it ended up to be a seminoma of the media-sternum, which is really, really unusual. But he got better and was able to graduate from the university."

At the clinic in Vinton, Harold sees 30 to 40 patients a day, everything from the very young to geriatric patients.

"I see a variety of cases, a lot of upper respiratory stuff, a lot of GI stuff," he said. "I do a lot of emergency room work. You see everything in the emergency room, as you know, heart attacks, surgical emergencies of all kinds.

"There are these codes that come in by ambulance. And it is hard to say how long the people have been without a heartbeat. A lot of those you can't save, but once in a while you get one that comes in with chest pain and your nose tells you it is a heart attack. But you have nothing else that documents that and you have to fight with the cardiologist.

"Well, one night we put this guy in the hospital and he didn't have any cardiac complaints at first. He just didn't feel good. And so we were getting him in bed and all of a sudden we were at the nurses station and we looked up at the monitor and he went into defib just while we were sitting there and watching. We ran down to his room and defibrillated him and he comes back. We saved his life. I have had that happen several times, situations like that. Most of them you can't save.

"There is this other case of a 44-year-old guy who was out hunting with his kids one Sunday morning. I happened to be on call when he came into the emergency room. He was having just left shoulder pain. He thought he pulled a shoulder muscle. Anyway I looked at him and he just looked terrible to me. He just had that funny look about him, one of those nondescript looks. It just looked like trouble was coming.

"So I did an EKG and he was having a heart attack. I called the cardiologist in Cedar Rapids. The guy is doing fine, I'm controlling his pain with nitro and morphine. So the cardiologist says give him TPA—an enzyme to dissolve a blood clot—so I gave him TPA and the helicopter shows up. He looked stable, he was talking and joking to the nurses and everybody. Well, we got him downstairs to go out to the helicopter pad and he goes into defib. Right there, on the way out.

"We got the defibrillator that was in the flight crew's sack but we couldn't get his rhythm stabilized. We shocked him and he came back and then he would go back into defib, back and forth, back and forth. I felt so bad about it because his wife was in the emergency room and I said, 'Well, you go down to St. Luke's Hospital and you meet your husband there.' So she took off before this happened. I was sitting there thinking, Jesus, this guy is going to die on me and I just told his wife that everything was OK. Anyway, we finally got him back. We used every drug in the book. Finally, beryllium, we used that and stabilized his heart rate and he got down to Cedar Rapids and they took him into the cath lab and I guess he would defib on and off in the cath lab. So anyway, Dr. Provany was taking care of him and he got him opened up and he has been doing fine ever since."

When I'd asked him all the questions I could think of, Harold and I went into an Italian restaurant, and sat at the bar for a while. We were like old warriors recalling the last 30 years and events and happenings and people we've known over the years and who have gone now. We laughed a lot and it was fun to be with him again. He is a very competent practitioner of medicine, actually. He is a good physician assistant.

He is "one of the good guys."

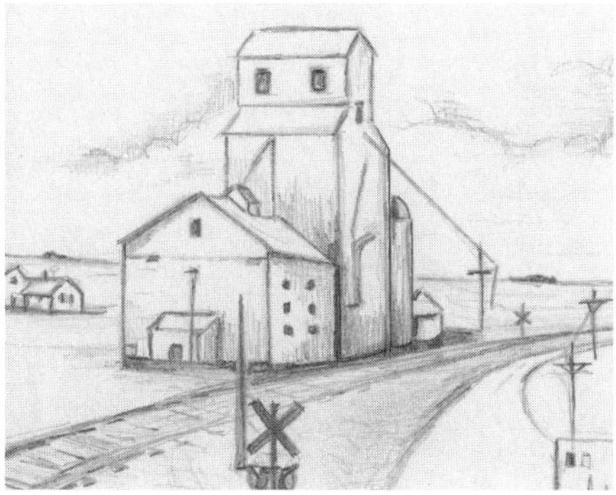

5

A Wonderful Lady

WHILE MEDEX GRADUATES like Harold Vanscoy proved their worth in the field as well as in demonstrating the value of the program that trained them, the Vietnam War was drawing to a close in the early 1970s, and with it the supply of newly returning independent-duty corpsmen. We were able to fill our first two classes with them, but in the third year we couldn't find enough students with just the right level of experience and medical background.

In truth, the MEDEX model left a few things to be desired. The most obvious was the disconnect between our graduates those first three years and the underserved areas in which we'd hoped to place them. Frankly, in many cases the placement was a mismatch. The students did fine, they learned what they needed to learn and did well with their preceptors. And they went on to solid careers in hands-on medicine. But getting them to commit to settling down in out-of-the way locales was just not a realistic expectation.

For the most part, these were men who had not only seen the horrors of war, but who already had seen much of the world and weren't really prepared to confine themselves to a remote corner of it for the rest of their working lives. It reminded me a little bit of the old song title "How ya gonna keep 'em down on the farm after they've seen Paree?"

There was another issue as well. Before the MEDEX students arrived, we received a grant from the U.S. Department of Labor to train the unemployed to become assistants to nurses, doctors and dieticians, etc. But that funding came loaded with restrictions, many of which made no sense to me. For instance, the time element: They said we had to complete our training in three months. But we had already boiled down 14 years' worth of knowledge into 18 months. Further cutting it to 90 days was insane. So we went ahead and trained five nurses—who were not unemployed—over a period of 18 months to become nurse practitioners.

Among other strange rules: they wouldn't let us pay for any consultants more than 100 miles away and, while we could use male models for male genital exams, we couldn't use female models. I saw such rules as bureaucratic nonsense and, to make a long story short, we ended up intentionally or, out of frustration, violating almost every rule they had. I did this under a precept I'd learned from my friend, Tom Clifford: it is easier to ask forgiveness than permission.

I had come to appreciate the value of that strategy over a long and valued friendship with Tom, whom I'd met on the handball courts at UND in the late 1950s. Tom was then the vice president of finance at the university. He was also a decorated U.S. Marine combat officer in the Pacific during World War II, an attorney, an accountant, and one of those rare individuals who was not only supremely self-confident but who regularly exercised an easy sense of humor. North Dakota politicians on both sides of the aisle counted Tom as a friend. And while Tom never made known to anyone his political party, both Democrats and Republicans were equally convinced that he was one of theirs.

That certainly didn't hurt when George Starcher, the UND president at the time, retired and a successor was sought. Tom fit the bill perfectly and during his tenure as president, his support and interference-running on behalf of our department meant the difference between success and failure.

The most significant aspect of that support came in the way Tom allowed the Department of Community Medicine complete discretion over the use of outside funding that came into the program. The standard rule at UND was that outside funding went directly into the state coffers. From there, under the state's annual budget, some of it flowed back to the university. At that point, under the university's budget, it was parceled out to various college needs and then, at last, to the originating department or program.

By the time that parcel got to the originating program it was considerably lighter than when it first arrived. But the idea of a state or university laying claim to a percentage of outside funding was and remains nothing new. It is done everywhere under the sanctioned procedure of labeling such percentages as necessary "educational costs."

We were really kind of an experimental program. Tom allowed us to expand as we saw fit and, for that, we needed all of our funding. As Tom put it to me, "You can't go begging to the university for more money because you are not going to get it." So we had to go out and get our own money, which we did and we took advantage of the "educational costs" game to circumvent the normal procedure. We even used some of it to build our lecture hall on the fourth floor of the School of Medicine building—finally giving the program a status of legitimacy.

Tom's standard approach as president was always hands-off. However, while he was never a micro-manager, his expectation that you would use that freedom of movement to grow and to succeed was resoundingly clear. A lot of people would say of Tom that he always gave you enough rope to hang yourself. Of course, if you knew your way around rope, you found you had nothing to fear, and your relationship with the president remained positive.

I had no trouble accepting that challenge from Tom, who was a champion competitor on the handball courts. But many others in the university resented it. Those were days when outside funding wasn't the norm and departments and programs were used to simply getting by on what the university budgeted. Tom liked to tell such people to use their initiative and find some funding and they'd get the same deal as we did. However, very few took that advice.

The system worked for us to the extent that I never once, in 28 years, had to ask my dean for any extra funding. In fact, one year the dean came to me and asked if we would loan him $100,000 to cover a budget shortfall. We did and the dean repaid it in the next quarter. Many years later, when there came a time when we lost all of our outside funding, we simply increased the size of the program and operated off of the increased tuition. Instead of calling it tuition, however, we again referred to it as "educational costs."

This was another source of resentment campus-wide. Normally, students paid tuition to the university, a portion of which was channeled back to the originating department. Again, Tom Clifford liked that we were a self-sufficient, successful program, and he didn't interfere with us. In the end we probably gave back to the university more than the university gave to us.

By the way, as soon as I retired—several years after Tom himself had retired—our training program was incorporated into the academic bowels of the university and the cost for training a student just about doubled. Everybody, particularly the dean's office, wanted a little piece of that money.

During that third year of our MEDEX Program, when we ran out of medics, we decided to fill some slots with local nurses who had shown interest in playing a more central role in health care delivery. Much of the credit behind this idea goes to Mickey Knutson, herself an excellent nurse and a very shrewd judge of talent.

Not only did she see nurses as providing an inexhaustible supply of students in future years, she also found a source of funding that made that strategy possible.

The need for new funding had become obvious. While we already had the Department of Labor grants, the feds were not thrilled at the way we ignored or worked around their numerous regulations. Ours had become a strained relationship and, coupled with the dearth of independent corpsmen, seemed destined for a divorce. Then Mickey persuaded Barbara Lee of the W.K. Kellogg Foundation to consider our program. It was an ideal match for Kellogg's stated philanthropic goal at the time to increase the number of nurses and health care administrators in the country.

Kellogg provided enough funding over the next 15 years that we no longer needed the troublesome grant from the Department of Labor. In fact, I was able to send back several hundred thousand dollars with a "thanks, but no thanks" letter.

There was one odd catch, however, to the initial Kellogg funding. Barbara Lee told Mickey that we would get the funding if—and only if—we agreed to train seven nurses in Iowa on behalf of an energetic nun named Sister Mary Brigid.

Calling her an energetic member of the Sisters of Mercy doesn't quite do her justice, however. When we met her in 1974, her list of accomplishments was stunning. She had already earned master's and Ph.D. degrees in nursing from the University of Iowa and had written four books on her order, the Sisters of Mercy.

She'd been head of the Department of Nursing and a professor at St. Ambrose College and Marycrest College in Davenport for 19 years. In 1974 she was vice president of the Iowa Hospital Association in Des Moines and held gubernatorial appointments to the Iowa Board of Nursing and to the Physician Assistants Board.

The sister was extremely well connected to the nursing and medical field not only in Iowa but across the Midwest. It was said that when one of her nurses or hospitals needed something all she had to do was twist the arm of one of her Irish Mafia connections in the medical world.

Whether Barbara Lee qualified as one of those or not, Sister Brigid and she were close. When our program came along, it seemed to them heaven-sent. Barbara was our contract officer with Kellogg and she was also the contract officer for Sister Brigid. It seemed like an odd arrangement until we saw the high quality of nurses Sister Mary Brigid sent to us. We ended up training seven of them at the start, and others over the years. Every one of them turned out fine. Sister Brigid even lined up doctor-preceptors to work with them. I'm told she did this by telling each of them—in her own version of making them an offer they couldn't refuse—"You will train these girls." And they all dutifully responded, "Yes, sister."

When Mickey and I went to Iowa to conduct site visits with those preceptors, Sister Brigid would drive us around the state. I remember well her driving us through Iowa and going through every possible red light she came to. Or so it seemed, because I remember thinking that we were never going to survive the whole damn trip. Often Sister Brigid would stay with us at a local hotel and even then she was full of energy. One night she was jumping rope in her room to stay fit.

Which reminds me of the story told to me by Linda Rubel and Ann Diehl, nurses who came through our program and two of those first seven sent by Sister Brigid. I interviewed both of them with their husbands one night in January 2000 in a Des Moines restaurant. During our dinner the topic naturally came around to Sister Brigid, whom Linda and Ann—and apparently all of the good sister's charges—called "Bridgy."

Linda recalled the time Bridgy went on an exercise kick:

"She said, 'I have to tell you girls. I decided I needed to get healthy so I am watching my diet and I am going to exercise class. Well, she said, I went out and they told us we had to have leotards. I didn't know what leotards were. I went to buy them and I certainly found out. I have never worn anything like a leotard but the woman leading the class said you will wear leotards. So I put on my leotards and the next thing she said was to sit on the floor. I said, my God, I have never sat on the floor in my life. But I sat on the floor and then she said, 'Spread your legs apart.' And, my God, they wouldn't come apart.'"

Ann had a tale to match.

"In Iowa," she said, " there are several farms where there are just acres of strawberries and acres of raspberries and you can go out and pick your own. I told Bridgy I was going to do this and she sort of invited herself along. So we pick up this nun, dressed in her full habit, and we go to the farm and the owner gives us this little basket and he explains: 'You pick a row and you stay on the same side of the row and you work it as far as you want to.' So Richard and I got our baskets and we start picking. And we heard some people talking and grumbling. And we looked up and people are pointing at a nun who is running around, skimming the ripe raspberries off the top of every bush. She is not walking a row as we were told to. She zigzagged all over. I mean, it is kind of hard to pretend you are not with a nun."

A side note about Linda and Ann: Not until they were accepted into the program—through Sister Mary Brigid's recommendation—and arrived in Grand Forks, did they tell anyone that they were sisters.

"When we applied," Linda told me, "we were both excited and then we said, 'Oh, oh, what if one of us makes it and the other one doesn't?' We were dreaming we both would. So we made a pact, whoever got it, the other would be happy and rejoice. Well, I got my acceptance in the mail and I called Ann and I was so excited and there was silence and she said, 'I didn't get one.' I began to cry and she began to cry and I said, 'Well I am not going then. I am just not going.' She said, 'Oh yes you are.' Then she got her acceptance in the mail the next day.

"But we never told anybody that we were sisters. We thought it would hurt our chances. Sister Mary Brigid didn't know that either. And when we all met, all the selected candidates for the first time in North Dakota, we said, 'Well, we need to tell you this so that you know it. We are sisters.' We got a blank look from everyone. They thought we were nuns. And then it finally connected."

It was that strange moment that started the whole business of medical extenders in Iowa. Sister Mary Brigid's nurses—who became nurse practitioners—really pioneered the whole thing.

During those first three years before we went exclusively with trained nurses as students, we learned an awful lot about our curriculum's needs and about some of the pitfalls and we became a little bit more sophisticated every year. Our program became strictly one of demand. If there was demand, we did the training.

If we didn't have the demand, we didn't do the training. Often our classes were 15 students. Sometimes, during our Kellogg years, they went up to a high of 30 students, usually including one or two from Iowa.

By the way, Sister Mary Brigid died just a year ago at the age of 93 in Aurora, Ill., where she'd joined the Sisters of Mercy 78 years earlier. In her obituary she was quoted as saying, "I had a wonderful life, now I'm ready to meet my God."

She was just a dynamo, a wonderful lady.

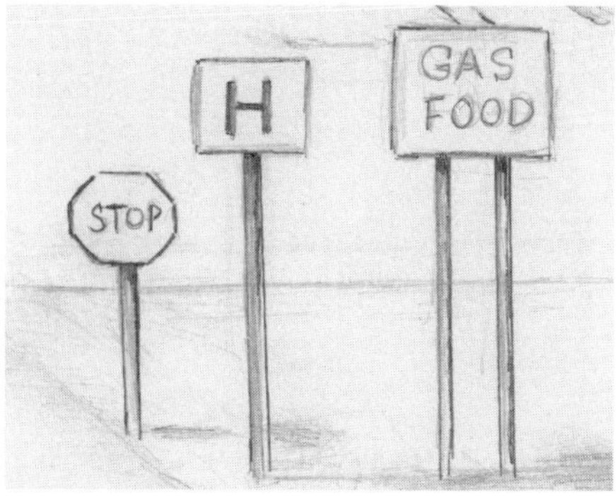

6

A Pugilistic Nose

In North Dakota, as in many Midwestern states, you will find people working hard in their regular daytime career jobs as bankers, teachers, lawyers and so forth, who, also work very hard at a part-time job. Perhaps "job" isn't the right word; it's more like an avocation. Or even a hobby. Or just something that is in your blood. I'm talking about farming.

If you were raised on a farm or in a home where a parent did part-time farming, it might seem natural that in your spare hours you'd find your relaxation by climbing onto your tractor and tilling the south 40. North Dakota has its share of those part-time farmers, but there are also men and women who didn't grow up with farmers, who nevertheless have taken to working the land with great enjoyment and industry.

Of course there are also those folks who did grow up with parent farmers who do not have it in their blood and who do not farm either full time, part time or anytime. I am one of those. In my defense, I will say that at least I gave it a long—and sobering—tryout before throwing up my hands in surrender.

For most of his adult life, my father was a teacher or a school administrator. But when he became the young superintendent of schools in Drayton in 1916, he and a couple of friends went in together on a three-quarter section of farmland. He formed what he called the Drayton Land Company and was extremely proud to be a landowner. He eventually bought out his partners and dabbled in farming in between running the Drayton schools and playing baseball for the town team. He never made much money in his farming and when he and my mother moved on to Groton, S.D., after World War I, he leased the land to Pete and Anna Helm. Curiously, one of Pete and Anna's future grandsons—Harold Helm—would one day become my son-in-law.

Groton is where my sister Barbara was born—and died only three days later. To bring my mother out of her depression, my dad booked passage in 1925 on the USS Roosevelt and they sailed to Europe for a tour of England, Holland and Germany. When they returned, my brother, the future radiologist, Herman Harrison Eelkema, was born. Meanwhile, my father, an erstwhile musician, started a marching band in the school where he and my mother taught. Ever industrious, he also began studying law through correspondence courses with a university in California.

The family moved briefly to Mankato, Minn., for another teaching job. The only event there of any import was the birth in 1930 of the previously mentioned Baby Boy Eelkema. Shortly after, the family moved to Iowa where my father had been accepted as a graduate student at the University of Iowa. I have only vague memories of Iowa City, where we lived until I was three years old. While there, my dad earned his Ph.D. in education, writing his thesis on the use of bonds to finance school buildings. That same year he got his law degree. He passed the bar in Iowa and then in Illinois, where the high school in the Cook County town of Proviso Township in Maywood, Ill., near Chicago, hired him as superintendent of schools.

We lived in Maywood, very close to the site of the 1933-34 Chicago World's Fair. I remember vividly walking to the fairgrounds and watching racecars doing daredevil stunts, like driving through fire. And I recall that the house my parents rented had no air conditioning, so in the summer we took all the mattresses downstairs where it was cooler.

During his time as superintendent, Dad got a bond issue passed for a large gymnasium on the east side of Proviso. This was the middle of the Great Depression and the only real construction jobs available were in the school system. Many of the school board members wanted to make sure their friends got employment, so the bids had to go out to their pals. There was an awful lot of under-the-table type activity and Dad was really under the gun to go along with it. But being as straight a man as he was, he didn't care for it, and soon was sending his resume out. He landed a superintendent's job in Duluth, Minn., hoping maybe it would be a better fit.

As it turned out, it wasn't. My father's various tenures as a school superintendent never lasted that long. The way school politics goes, someone was always getting mad at him and he was always on one hot seat or another. In Duluth, he ran into trouble with a hostile board of education. When he came to town in 1936 he was forced to close schools and lay off teachers. He quickly became the bad guy. He used to come home at night and complain of migraine headaches. He and Mom would have lengthy talks about the job and I knew that there was a lot of tension.

To get away from the hostility, he began making trips back to Drayton, working his land and buying up a little more here and there. As time went on, he was spending more time at the farm than in school work.

On the positive side of the ledger, it was in Duluth that my dad bought a home for the first time in his life. Built by some early Duluth millionaires, it was a beautiful, old three-story house overlooking Lake Superior. All the wood was mahogany and there was silk wallpaper in the living and dining rooms. There were servants' quarters and bell ropes to summon them. My father bought it from a widow who owned an electric car; the purchase included a building out back equipped with electrical chargers. There were plenty of nooks and crannies in that house, even a crawl space under the third floor where my brother and I loved to explore.

Duluth is a very long and narrow town—18 miles from east to west—built on a hill overlooking Lake Superior. I can still hear the toot of the foghorns on the ore boats as they came into port. Duluth was a steel town in those days. Most people worked in the mills, turning all of that iron ore, brought in by boat, into steel. Most of the houses were pretty much alike. In my early Duluth days I remember playing at Leif Erickson Park. Very much an immigrant's town, its citizens came from Norway, Sweden, Canada and Greece.

I started first grade in Duluth and soon met a best friend for life in Dave Beamer. He's now a retired Presbyterian minister, a very tender, caring guy. There was another long-time pal, a kid named Sherman Winthrop, whose parents owned the Ideal Grocery. A kid named Hal Ryan, lived next door to us in Duluth. In the basement, Hal's grandma made soap using grease and lard. His dad was a lawyer and he'd sit on the porch with us and keep telling us say how important it was to have an education. He was always trying to convince us to become lawyers.

In the meantime, Dave, Sherm and I loved to do things together, mostly athletics of some form. We'd go to an empty lot and let the word get around that we were choosing up sides for a game. Of course, you never wanted to be the last person picked.

We'd play touch football and baseball, kick the can, basketball. I can't remember not being outside and not playing. There was no reason to stay inside, even in wintertime. In the snowy season, my mother sewed leather onto the seat of my pants and on the knees and we'd go out and slide down the snowbanks. We wore knickers then and called them turd catchers.

When Sherm, Dave and I went to middle school, we all wanted to play basketball and to make the team, which we did. We'd get up early and practice basketball before class started. I played sports all through middle school and high school and had several offers for a small-college football scholarship.

My folks gave a lot of dinner parties, something that was expected of the superintendent of schools. Lots of times they would empty out the house and the dining room and bring in chairs and tables from the school system. And they'd have meals for teachers and administrators and we were expected to disappear.

My mother always looked elegant. She had long black hair. She would either braid it or she would put it up into a bun. She played the role of the dutiful wife of an administrator, but she was very much an educated woman. She was very literate, a member of the Book of the Month club who always had a book in her face, reading. She was impeccable in her English and she would not let any of us end a sentence with a preposition. Or say "ain't." Or be anything but appropriate.

She was a fun-loving person, and so was my dad when it comes right down to it. They both liked to laugh. When we ate dinner, however, he'd put the dinner plates in front of him. My mother would come out of the kitchen with the meal—the beef or the potatoes and beets or whatever. And he would serve it up and pass the plate. And we were expected to eat what he served up on the plate. And, believe me, we did. His word was iron.

Years later, when my kids and I visited my parents in Duluth, the kids were shaking in their boots because they knew they had to eat what was on their plate. We used to call him "Old blood and guts" or "Papasall," for "Papa is all."

My mother kind of let him run the household, but she ended up usually being the boss in her own inimitable way. When it came right down to making decisions she was the one who made them. I know she used to kick him in the shins under the table once in a while.

Over the years my father got disenchanted with Roosevelt. He'd complain that he was trying to pack the Supreme Court and trying to pass a lot of social programs that my dad objected to. My mother always thought differently. When they went to the polls I think they canceled each other out.

Both my parents were musically inclined and they had this great notion in those days that I would become a dancer. They bought me a pair of black patent leather shoes and put taps on them. They took me down to a Christmas program at the Palmer

House hotel in Chicago and had me go up on the stage to tap dance. I had no idea how to tap dance. Let me tell you, I was not a musician. I could not keep time and I was pretty hopeless. I think I was a disappointment to my parents. Everybody wants their kids to be something.

When I washed out on the dance floor they pushed me toward music. We had a piano that my mother played. My father played trumpet and violin and later the mandolin. We used to sit around the piano while mother played. We'd sing all the old songs like "Yes, we have no bananas." They wanted me to be able to play the piano, but I couldn't keep a tune. Two blocks from our house was a conservatory of music run by Catholic sisters. I went there once a week for two years for piano lessons. The nun finally told my folks it was a total waste of money.

My music career was sinking fast, but not quite over. In school I heard that if you took band you didn't have to take music. Does that even make sense? Anyway, I signed up for band, which pleased my father. Of course, I had no idea what I'd do. At first I took home a big bass, but it was too heavy. I tried all the horns, but I couldn't even make a noise out of them. My dad changed his violin strings so I could play it left-handed. That was a total waste of time.

I finally degenerated down to drums. Unfortunately I wasn't that handy with the drumsticks. So they put me on the bass drum, but I couldn't even make an after-beat. The band director used to come back to where I sat with the drum and hit my head with a baton. He'd say, "Every time I hit your head, you hit the drum." I couldn't even do that. He finally ended up sending me on errands. I was tone deaf, timing deaf and just didn't have it. I did, however, write a composition for my English teacher about my musical career and for that I got an A+.

Whether it was something like dancing or piano lessons, Dad was always trying to improve us to the point of perfection. It never seemed to work with me. One day my brother and I were playing and he pushed me down the basement stairs. I landed on my nose and broke it. My Dad wanted my nose to be perfect, so he took me to a specialist who put a bandage on it. But all attempts by my father to make me pretty were negated. Playing football for Central High School in Duluth and the University of Minnesota in Duluth, I broke my nose five times. I ended up needing a sub-mucous resection and to this day have somewhat of a pugilistic nose.

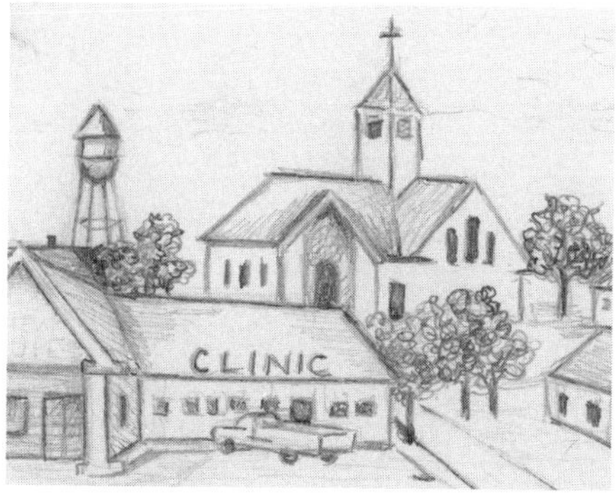

7

The Only Drugstore in Town

NOVEMBER 5, 1999

I AM ON U.S. 93, about 85 miles north of Las Vegas, heading for Alamo, Nev. I'm going to meet Geraldine Perkins at the Del Pueblo Restaurant at 12 noon. It is 11:35 a.m. now and I am not sure exactly where Alamo is. I am still on a very lonesome road going up there. The highway cuts through the Pahranagat Valley, with the Sheep Mountain Range on either side. It's part of a national wildlife refuge and it's mostly desert. According to my map, just a few miles up the road from Alamo is the Extra Terrestrial Highway. It goes west through Area 51, where the U.S. Air Force is supposed to have conducted experiments on aliens from outer space. I almost feel like an alien myself, stranded on some empty planet.

I remember a site visit I conducted up here years ago. I was supposed to pick up Geraldine—everyone calls her Geri—in Alamo and then drive her over to Caliente, which is two mountain ranges east of where I am now. But those instructions weren't on my site-visit sheet. So I drove all the way to Caliente, 75 miles east of Alamo, and not knowing Geri was waiting for me to pick her up. One of the things that she was looking forward to was driving in my air-conditioned car, which she didn't have, and it was about 120 degrees in the shade. So she had to take her very rudimentary and primitive car without air-conditioning and sweat it out.

I just passed a lone highway sign and all it said was "North." It is sort of nice to know that I am still going north. And there is water up here and they are starting to get some trees. Beautiful, beautiful trees up ahead, so it is kind of an oasis town, I guess. The leaves are just starting to turn.

I just spotted a 911 number on the side of the road that says, "Emergency Medical Services." Now I see a water tower up on the hill and it says, "Alamo." It is a huge tank with the elevation written on it: 3,450 feet above sea level. There is a sign for the airport, but it's not much more than a lone runway. Just passed Lamb Boulevard. I suspect that sheep are big up here in the Sheep Range.

I'm in town now and all I can see is a gas station with a great big sign that says, "Restaurant." No other sign, just "Restaurant." So I suspect I have to get further into town to find the Del Pueblo.

I just stopped and asked someone where the Del Pueblo was and he said it was back on the road about a quarter-mile. That is just where I came from. I think I was supposed to turn at the Chevron station. Then the guy starts yelling at me. "Say, you are holding up traffic." The town has a population of 1,000 and so far I've seen about two other cars, and now I'm in a traffic jam.

So there it is. Under the sign that says, "Restaurant." I guess everybody in town knows that it is the Del Pueblo. I am the only one who didn't know.

Geri is the mother of six children and she is very much a Mormon. She moved her family here from another nearby small town when she started as a physician assistant.

"I raised my family here," she told me, "so I am happy."

That, of course, is the ideal situation: to be married to the area and love it.

One of the first things I asked was if she thought a man could do the job as well as a woman. I'd forgotten that before she was posted here, the town had a male physician assistant who, like

Geri, was married and had a family.

"What prompted him to leave?"

"Well, none of them ever stay very long," she said, "because they weren't born and raised here. They have no roots. So they just stay until a better job comes a long."

Geri was a registered nurse before she came to UND for her PA training. She was friends with the PA in Alamo immediately before her, who was pregnant. She urged Geri to get into our program and come back to Alamo and share the practice with her.

"But by the time I graduated, she had moved," said Geri. "She just left me with the whole thing."

I am now sitting here in the Alamo Clinic after a quick lunch. Geri is very conscientious. She says she had to be back at the clinic at 1 p.m. because she didn't want to keep any patients waiting. I just read in a book that the unspoken word is an essential part of a conversation. It has to do with the way people inflect, given the ambience of a particular area, that is something you can't hear on a phone or with telecommunications. When you walk into a clinic you can actually feel either the acceptance or the rejection. Here, I feel the acceptance, even though the clinic is nothing more than a double-wide trailer.

The waiting room is a narrow hallway and patients talk to each other like long-lost buddies. There is an old carton full of kids' toys, beanie babies and things like that. There is a computer here in the office, but it doesn't look like it's getting a lot of action. On the wall I see Geri's American Nurses' Credentialing Center certificate, her diploma from the University of North Dakota, her baccalaureate degree in nursing from the University of Utah, her Nevada State Board of Nursing license and also her physician assistant certification from the National Commission of Certification of Physician Assistants. Oh, and her certificate from the Nevada State Board of Pharmacy.

On the office table is a book called "Spanish Made Simple" and I think maybe they have a fair number of Hispanics in the area. On her desktop is kind of a mini-library: Nelson's Text of Pediatrics, Primary Care of Women, Sport Injuries, Atlas of Emergency Procedures, Guide to Physical Examination, Current Medical Diagnosis and Treatment, Emergency Medicine, Diagnosis and Training of Treatment of Communicable Common Kids' Diseases, Clinical Dermatology, Dictionary of Medicine and Nursing.

So far, since lunch, Geri took a Pap smear; gave a flu shot and a tetanus shot; explained to a prospective emergency medical technician (EMT) what the test to get certified would be like, and encouraged and counseled a young woman who had tried to commit suicide—all in a space of about a half an hour. It looks like she has quite a loyal following.

"I feel that I can make a difference," Geri told me over lunch. "I have enjoyed teaching the EMTs so that they can do more. Before I started doing that they would just load people up and go. Now they can stop and take care of patients."

What a wonderful, wonderful statement. That is an attitude that unfortunately is little practiced in the big city.

Geri's hours are 9 to 5, and the clinic is open five days a week. She does a lot of infant care but she also does the vaccinations and the well-child check-ups and so forth. Not surprisingly, she does a lot of women's health too. Pelvic exams and Pap smears. A mobile mammogram unit comes in twice a year.

There is no X-ray facility here, nor a lab, although she is able to do urine dips and pregnancy tests. She sends all her lab work to a private pathology lab in Las Vegas. A currier picks up all the blood samples and Pap smears from the clinic at 4:30 p.m. every day and takes them 90 miles south to Vegas. At 4 a.m. or even earlier they will fax the results to the clinic so, when she gets there at 9 a.m., they are already there—Sunday, holidays and everything.

She does have an electrocardiogram (EKG) machine and was trained in its use by Dr. Phillips in Eureka. I asked her what she would do if someone came in with a heart attack.

"I would do the definitive care to stabilize them, call the Flight for Life helicopter out of Las Vegas and then the ambulance, which picks them up and meets the flight—unless I decide to keep the patient right here because he is unstable. In that case they will come and pick him up."

She doesn't really have a bed at the clinic for that, just the two rooms, one she uses as a regular patient room and one that she calls her "little emergency room" which is always ready for the unexpected.

"I have some exciting things which drive up every now and then," she said. "A guy came running in and I was at lunch and the nurse was still here and he said this woman is having a baby outside. So she went outside and could see the baby crowning and came back inside to get supplies and just then I drove up and so I grabbed some gloves and we went out there and the baby's head came out and I couldn't get it out. The baby had been in and out for about 20 minutes but I could not get it out. I had never intubated a newborn before, so that was a first. But I did it and by then Flight had gotten here. We called them immediately of course. So it is not all colds and sore throats."

I have noticed a pharmacy certificate in her office. She is a pharmacist as well as a medical provider.

"You are the only drugstore in town?"

"There is nobody else."

If she runs out of a drug she calls it in to a pharmacy in Caliente, 75 miles away.

"I buy my sulfa in bottles of a thousand and I buy my biaxin in bottles of 60. I don't use much tetracycline but I keep it stocked because there are some vaginal infections. I buy my amoxicillin 40 bottles at a time. Most of the medicine I buy is already prepackaged in bottles of 30 so I just have to dispense one bottle."

Geri and her husband, who is retired (she refers to him as Perkins), live on a 20- acre farm about four miles outside of town. They lease out the pasture to those who want to put their cows there. She says they usually spend their vacations visiting some or all of their six grown children who are scattered all over. I asked her if they had a camper and she was quick to say "no."

"I don't consider that a vacation. My husband would, but I don't. My idea of a vacation is to stay in a motel and eat in restaurants. I don't like camping out."

When she retires, she and her husband plan on going out as

Mormon missionaries somewhere and doing something. They are really interested in making a difference in the world, which I think represents the motivation of a lot of our students.

One of the things that Geri was worried about is that her life was so simple and so unexciting that it would probably not go down well in a narrative as being anything particularly good. She doesn't think of herself as being important or even significant enough that other people would want to read about what her job is out here and what she does.

But I beg to differ on that. I think the world needs to know what the Geri Perkinses of the world do. She is really a jack-of-all-trades. She does everything. That is how it is when you are living in Alamo, Nev. Professionals like Geri are people who are extremely confident, intelligent, well-trained. They have come through our program as adult-learners and they have a lot of offer. And they do it because it is a calling, a passion.

They are living in an area that a doctor wouldn't come near. Most doctors specialize anyway. They don't know what the hell is going on half the time.

They are as scared as could be to be out here alone. They would be here shaking in their boots about some of the things that have to be done. When she takes a vacation, the pediatrician from Caliente will come over maybe a couple days a week. Otherwise they close the clinic. Everybody in town knows that Geri is gone.

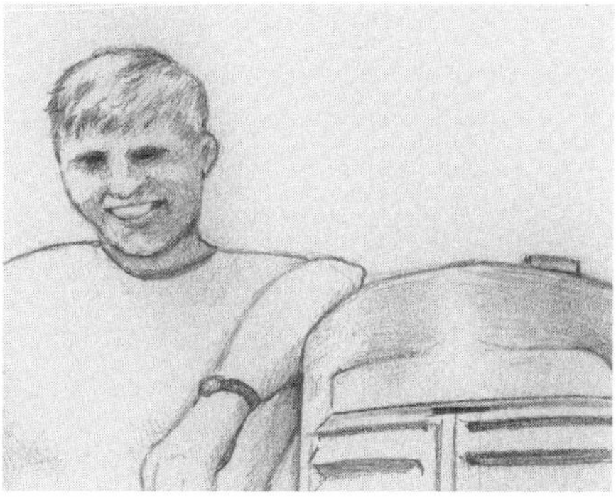

8

The Hayseed

On Sundays during those Duluth days my father would take us all on a drive into the country. By that time there were five of us, including my sister, Ruth, who was born just after we moved there. One December Sunday we were out driving in my father's new 1941 Studebaker Commander when President Roosevelt came on and started talking about the day that would go down in infamy. As it did to so many around the world, that moment would change our lives.

That summer, in 1942 when I was 12, I went with my dad up to the farm in Drayton. He was raising potatoes and we lived in a boarding house while my mother stayed back in Duluth.

There was a farmer in town who needed some help harvesting his crops. His son was in the service. During the war all the young men were gone. We who were too young to go to war were expected to take on the role of a man very early in life. When I think of 12-year-olds now, even 15-year-olds, they are treated like kids and adolescents and not given much responsibility. In those days they expected us to grow up a little faster than they do now.

So that farmer hired me and paid me $5.50 a day, including my room and board. He had a combine and a wagon in the field. He would empty his grain into the wagon and I'd shovel it out of the wagon into his '37 Ford truck. Then I'd take the truck down to the grain elevator. I was 12 and, of course, had no driver's license. But that's what I did all day.

One time I got up to the elevator and they didn't have any more room. So I went to another elevator not too far from the farm. And I heard the guy there talking to one of his helpers and I knew what he was up to. I brought the truck up and I told the guy to get his hands off the scale. And he said, "You smart aleck whippersnapper. For that I won't empty your truck." I was trying to protect the farmer from getting cheated. So I called the farmer and he said take it into Auburn and I did. But none of them had any room. I ended up late at night taking the truck back home. And in the morning I was stuck shoveling it off into a small hole in the granary.

It got to be a pretty lonely summer. But a man driving a refurbished old hearse filled with dogs came through town one day. The guy was selling them and I looked in the back and there was a black cocker spaniel looking right at me, wagging his tail. I said I'd sure like to see that one. And he started licking my face and I knew I didn't have any right to do it but I said I'd sure like this one. How much? And he said five bucks and I'll even throw in a collar and leash. I said, "Well, I shouldn't do it, but I'll take it."

I couldn't take it back to the boarding house. I was afraid Dad would make me give it back. So a friend in the Drayton creamery took it overnight. But the dog ate all the ice cream cones, so I couldn't keep it there anymore. There was a small shed behind the boarding house so I stuck my new dog, Skipper, out there. That night, Dad kept saying, "Isn't there a dog barking out there?" I said, "Oh no." Well, he found out I had the dog, but he accepted it. Pretty soon he was teaching the dog all kinds of tricks. In German. But the dog slept with me and I had him from the time I was 12 until I was 21.

That fall when the potatoes came in there was talk about an

early frost. I remember the guy in charge wanted to finish off the spuds before the frost and he said, "Time-and-a-half for overtime past midnight." I wouldn't think that was so bad but the guy who was the boss happened to be my dad. When I think about it now I think, Oh my God. I'd already worked since ten o'clock in the morning.

By 1943, Dad was having a lot of trouble with Duluth's newly elected school board and he wasn't happy. He applied to the Army for a commission and they made him a major. Then they sent him for training to Charlottesville, Va. He got very lonely down there and we went to visit him, the three kids and my mother. She started out driving but her hands locked up on the steering wheel and she had trouble prying them off. My brother and I took turns driving the rest of the way, not knowing then that my mother's hand problem was the first vestige of Parkinson's disease, which would one day take her life.

My father mustered out of the Army in 1945 and he knew he couldn't go back to Duluth anymore. He spent a lot of time sending out resumes for administrative school work to just about every place in the country. I've got copies of all his applications. He was soon past 50 and that pretty much meant the end of his work-life as an administrator. They all wanted a young, vigorous 40-year-old to come in and work miracles in their school system.

But he still had the land in Drayton and he decided he was going to make a go of it there. He had about 3,000 acres. He was quite proud of that. When he died he was a millionaire on paper. But he was always cash-poor. That's what farmers are: land-rich and cash-poor.

Not long after he mustered out, my father took me up to Drayton and we refurbished the old house on the farm. He and my mother had kept the house in Duluth, where she remained during these post-war, North Dakota adventures. She refused to come up from Duluth until the Drayton farmhouse had running water and a bathroom. Eventually she did move up and they used the farmhouse from April or May until November. In the winter they both went to Duluth. One year, they went south, but they never liked it.

So they continued to stay north for the winter.

We had three cows to milk on the farm and my brother, Dad
 and I would come home at night and sometimes we would be late. The cows would jump the fence and come over to the front porch and go, "Moooo." And my Dad would say, "Who is going to milk the cows tonight?" Of course I would usually lose because I was the youngest. So I would just rattle the pails, jump the porch, go into the barn and milk those suckers. I don't think anybody realizes that they become pets.

Drayton, by the way, was where I had my first drink. The municipal liquor store was in the courthouse which was also the jail. And the man who sold me my first bottle of booze, peppermint schnapps, was the chief of police. I was 15. He said, "Old enough to work, old enough to drink." Dumb me, I thought if it was peppermint schnapps Dad wouldn't smell it on me. Only thing is, I came home and parked the car at an angle. He knew right away I had done something drastic.

Making a living off of the land is not an easy thing to do. Which is why my father decided to try hiring ourselves out to farmers who didn't have harvesting equipment. Some of our equipment was pretty rudimentary, so Dad bought two Massey-Harris combines. He had a brand-new Studebaker truck and a used 48 International. He had two hired men, both bachelors and his two sons.

He decided to take everything down South, looking for people who needed combine work. Wheat was maturing fast. So we headed for the first places we could get work. That was in Mount Vernon and Belleview, Kan. We didn't have any money so we slept in the back of the truck. Sometimes we'd sleep on the grain, sometimes in a sleeping bag on the hard truck bed. I got tired of sleeping in the truck and started sleeping on the ground. But I'd wake up with a headache. But when you're young you do those kind of things. And it's exciting.

We went to other towns in Nebraska and then up to South Dakota and pretty soon we got regular customers. We went down every year into the mid-1950s. Dad kept upgrading his equipment and the operation got pretty sophisticated after a while. It certainly saved the farm.

In the summer of 1948, after I'd graduated from Duluth's Central High School, I was still working on the farm. We had spuds again and it was raining all fall. My dad was putting me to work felling trees and I decided I didn't like any of that stuff anymore. So I called up my pal, Screech Wilson, and I said, "Let's go to California." I hitchhiked to Duluth and looked at used car lots. I found a '32 Plymouth for $89. It was four-cylinder, it had floating power, hydraulic brakes and four suicide doors. We even got insurance on it through Screech's dad.

We drove through Grand Forks and I called on a pay-phone and told my dad I was going to California. He says, "No, you're not." I said, "Yeah, we'll call you when we're out there." So we headed out with a great deal of hope and not very much money.

We averaged about 40 miles an hour. The car didn't have a proper gas gauge and in the middle of a hot day near the California-Nevada border we started on a 17-mile uphill climb. Three-quarters of the way up we ran out of gas. We had to back all the way down that hill and fill it up again.

By the time we hit California, the engine was going back and forth and the exhaust system was hitting the frame, going bang, bang, bang. We got to Los Angeles to where my cousin lived and we spent most of our time tearing apart that motor. He gave me ten bucks and another cousin gave me some cans of Dinty Moore's Beef Stew and we started out to go home. We'd hardly seen anything of California.

Between Barstow and Needles we heard a big bang and I could see oil on the running board and I knew we were in trouble. I drove up to a gas station and the guy there felt bad for us and he gave us $18 bucks for the car. We took all our belongings and went down to the train yard and climbed onto a gondola car. By the time we got off that train in Winslow, Ariz., we were so dirty and so black that when we went to a gas station they kicked us out.

We started hitchhiking into Tucumcari, N.M., and the cops locked us up for vagrancy. That night in the jail cell I wondered if we'd ever get out of that place. They let us out in the morning and we promised to take the first bus out of town. But we went to the eastern part of town and started hitchhiking again. We got picked up by a guy in a ten- gallon hat driving a convertible Cadillac. He was drunk, full of beer, and he took us into Amarillo, Tex. We were lucky to be alive.

We finally got home. I was 15 pounds lighter. Believe it or not, my folks were glad to see me. Probably ready to kill me, as well. Anyway there wasn't a wheel turned the whole three weeks we were gone, so I didn't get out of any work. We still had to harvest the potatoes. That's the year I started at University of Minnesota, Duluth. Because I was in such good shape they recruited me to play football. I played linebacker and center on offense.

In those days, between 1948 and 1952, football players didn't have a lot of safety equipment. About half the team's helmets had nose- and face-guards in them and half the team didn't. I was one of the lucky ones who had a guard. But not so lucky in what I did with it. One night, it was really cold and were playing St. Olaf College in Northfield, Minn. I was playing linebacker. We recovered a fumble so I came out and I threw my helmet on the ground and then, all of a sudden, we fumbled again and I had to run back onto the field. I couldn't find my helmet so I picked up somebody's helmet without the guard and on the first play I got kicked in the face and spit out my front teeth.

Well, I ended up marrying the dental assistant. I was only 20 years old. I had a '38 Plymouth and we had all our possessions, including wedding gifts, in the back seat when we headed for Drayton. Our honeymoon was going to the farm. The first night we stayed at Curly's cabin in Grand Rapids, Minn. In the morning we found the keys still in the car door. I wasn't too excited.

The next year my dad gave me 160 acres—one quarter section of land—to farm. I raised potatoes and flax. It was initially a wet year. I hadn't even gotten the last of the flax seed in before the first of it came up. When flax comes up, it blooms in blue. When you see it from a distance you think it's a big lake. It looked beautiful. The only problem was there wasn't a drop of rain on that land after it bloomed. The heads didn't fill out and I got a total of three bushels an acre, which isn't enough to buy a decent meal.

The potatoes, however, promised to be a real money-maker. Dad had put in 50 acres the year before and he'd cleared $5,000 which, in my mind, was an awful lot of money. But I couldn't afford to hire anybody to help with the planting.

I got a good stand of potatoes and had enough rain. I didn't have any storage facility so I had to sell them in what was called "field run." By then I was an accomplished sewer of potato sacks. I hired transient people to pick the potatoes. They put them in 100-pound sacks and left them for me to sew. I later went back with a truck and picked those hundred pound suckers up. Talk about work. I sold them field run at 70 cents a hundred. The way I counted and paid the pickers: I gave each one a gunny sack. Once they had 100 gunny sacks done they would come back for more. I paid them on the basis of sacks. Later on I found a lot of empty sacks back in the field. They were cheating me and I was essentially paying double. Not a good thing.

When I finished and got my expenses paid, I probably made $50 on the potatoes. I figured my time was worth about three cents an hour. Farming was in my blood but I didn't win on the first crop. It's like when you go to the racetrack for the first time and you win the first race and you're stuck for life. Well, I didn't win at farming.

But I still hadn't quite admitted to myself that farming wasn't for me. I took a lot of odd jobs, working as a cook and a cooking utensil salesman. I went back to school that summer and fall and took some animal husbandry courses and applied to veterinary school at the University of Minnesota. When they interviewed me they asked me why I wanted to become a vet. I said, well, I needed a vocation so I could make some money to go back and buy the farm. They accepted me because I probably answered it so honestly. I was really fortunate in that I got a scholarship through the whole four years of vet school.

During one of our early classes that first year, we took histology and were given a microscope. We were supposed to take it apart and identify all the pieces. Some people had trouble taking the eyepiece off. Well, I never went out to the south or west 40 without pliers. I still had a pair in my back pocket. So I pulled them out and started helping people unscrew the scope. I was known after that as "the hayseed with the pliers."

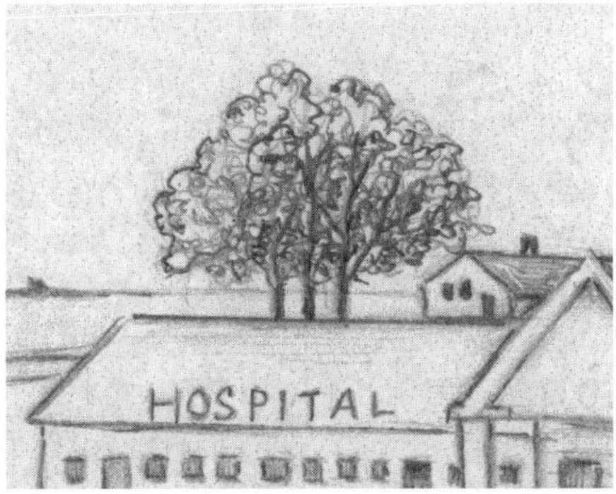

9

The Four Hundred

IN YOUR FIRST year as an official veterinarian, you learn what you can't learn in a classroom. Out in the field you really have to know what you're doing. But if you don't, it's best to keep your mouth shut and your eyes and ears open.

To wit: I got my first job out of veterinary school with an established vet in Valley City, N.D. The day I got there, my new partner said, "I'm going on vacation." He went up to Rocky Mountain Park in Manitoba for two weeks and left me all alone. I didn't know where anything was and I just had to shift for myself. During those two weeks I got seven horse calls. I figured my new partner didn't like horses and didn't want to go out on horse calls. So he saved them up for me.

I wasn't what you'd call an expert on horses—I wasn't an expert on anything at that point. But I knew enough to lead them out of the barn before I examined them. And three out of the seven actually collapsed and died on me.

They were 24- and 25-year-old nags but I was just mortified. I thought maybe I could have done something to help them a little bit. I did postmortems on a couple of them. One simply suffered a heart attack. One of them had a twisting of the bowel. So they had reasons to die. But I figured that was the end of it for me.

Since most of the action for a large-animal vet comes in the morning or at night, there wasn't a heck of a lot to do in the middle of the day. Once in while I'd go down to the Chevrolet dealer and sit on the couch in the waiting area and watch the new Chevrolets coming in. That qualified as excitement in Valley City. But during those first two weeks I overheard a conversation in the dealer's waiting room that perked up my ears.

Two men were talking about the new veterinarian in town. The one man said, "You know, this guy is so smart he can look into the eyes of a horse and he can tell when it's gonna die." It was a remark I wasn't really expecting, but after silently laughing to myself, I felt pretty good about it. I guess that's what you'd call unintended consequences.

Veterinary medicine, as it turned out, was a very good foundation for a public health doctor—because everything in veterinary medicine is public health. We had more virology in veterinary school than I had a few years later in medical school. That's because if you're a farmer or rancher and you wait for one of your animals to get sick, you're too late. The only way to be cost-effective in raising large animals and meat animals is to practice preventive medicine. It's too expensive, otherwise, to treat a chronic condition in a cow. If you told a farmer how much it costs, that cow would be sent to slaughter. So as a veterinarian, you're doing lots of immunizations for preventive stuff. Keeping the herd healthy for the farmer and the public is the name of the game.

While there's a lot to be said for spending money to prevent disease versus spending it on treating disease after the fact, in human medicine the focus we have and the expenditures we make are usually after the fact. Usually it's crisis care, when good, solid preventive medicine would have been more cost-effective—and life-supporting. The trouble is, it's very hard for a doctor to get reimbursed for practicing preventive medicine in humans. We tend to glorify and reward physicians who concentrate on crisis care. You're seeing these huge, huge salaries now for neurosurgeons and cardiovascular surgeons—not that they're not doing great work. But their narrow focus means they will see in the course of their careers patients numbering in the thousands—whereas public health people may actually save millions.

When I think back to those early days in veterinary school, it's not horses or medicine I'm remembering, but something much more mundane. I think I've slept on just about every possible bed known to man during my 81 years, but when Lois and I first got married and moved down to St. Paul, Minn., we came upon some of the worst beds known to man.

We were in the Twin Cities of Minneapolis and St. Paul because that is the home of the University of Minnesota's veterinary school. In that first year we rented a small apartment by the week in a place where we shared the refrigerator and bathroom with four or five other couples. Did I say it was very small?

The bed in the room was called a Murphy bed. When not in use, you lifted the end and it sprang back to its little hiding place in the wall. When you pulled it out from the wall it sat high on the feet and on the head and sagged in the middle almost like a hammock. In order to go to the bathroom or even the kitchen, you had to get out of the bed and move it back into the wall so you could get by. It wasn't pretty.

We got our name into the university housing office and we were able to move into a trailer. Did I say it was small? The trailer had a studio couch. When you opened it up, the one side was lower than the other side. There was quite a space in between the two sides and it was not easy to sleep on.

Eventually we got into what they called an expandable trailer—a tad bigger, though there really was nothing big about it at all. They made the beds with 2-by-4s and when you got in it everything sank right in the middle. Not an easy bed to sleep in. Some of our friends came along and looked at our bed and they felt really sorry for us and gave us an old brass bed. But it was so hard; it felt like you were sleeping high above the floor. You sat down and there was no give.

When our first daughter, Susan, was born in July 1952 we were eligible to move up into the more official student housing barracks where we had our own indoor facilities. But we also got a Hollywood bed which was just a mattress and springs. It sat on some very shaky legs, one of which broke soon after we moved in. I propped it up with Reader's Digests condensed books. And when the books fell off, then the bed fell off too. Luckily, when you're young you can put up with those kinds of things.

Actually, in terms of beds, the best one I slept in during veterinary school was a hospital bed, perhaps the only advantage to falling victim to a disease found in both humans and animals and known by a half-dozen names.

In the summers of my first three years in vet school we went out to various counties in Minnesota and tested animals for tuberculosis and something known as brucellosis. It was named after a British doctor named David Bruce who had been studying an illness that sprang up in Malta during the Crimean War in 1854. Until Bruce came along and linked it to an organism—dramatic stuff for nineteenth-century medicine—it had been known as Mediterranean fever and sometimes Crimean fever.

Ten years later a Danish veterinarian named Bernard Bangs found the specific organism behind the disease and it became known as Bangs. But about five years after that a Maltese doctor figured out that the primary source of the organism was unpasteurized milk. His name was Themistocles Zammit and, logically, one would assume the disease would become Zammit's disease. Instead, medical people began calling it Malta fever. At least Zammit got a knighthood out of it.

What I got was a miserable few weeks in a hospital and a major lesson about hygiene in the field. In cattle, Bangs—what we called it then—is connected to an infection that leads to an aborted fetus. I remember one time out in the Polk County area around Crookston, Minn., we saw a cow that had just aborted. I was testing it and the afterbirth was getting in my coveralls and I was wiping my face. Within two to three weeks after that I came down with a flaming case of Bangs. (Although, to confuse the issue even more, in humans it is known as undulant fever for the varying spikes in temperature.) By the time I went to the hospital I had already taken my own blood and checked the serology and found it to be a definitely positive. There happened to be a doctor in the area named Wesley Spinks who was treating people for undulant fever, with combinations of aureomyacin and streptomyacin. We started on that and I was feeling a lot better after three weeks.

Other than being in a decent bed for those weeks, there was one more positive offshoot of Bangs for me. I started reading seriously for the first time in my life. I read the whole volume of Lloyd C. Douglas's "Dr. Hudson's Secret Journal." I also found a whole pile of A.J. Cronin's novels about physicians in small towns. Then I got and read the entire set of Winston Churchill's history of World War Two. After that, I was hooked for life as an ardent devotee of reading.

I was not a good note-taker in vet school. One winter on a cold, snowy, icy day when I was just coming back from class, the wind got ahold of my notebook and scattered the papers everywhere. I lost a semester's worth of notes. But I had a good friend named Bob Caldwell who had been in the war and who played drums. He also took wonderful notes. He lent me his notebook and I learned how to outline and put down the important points. I was forever grateful for his assistance. After that I did very well with a 3.8 grade point average in my final two years.

In fact, I took some night school courses in English Constitutional history. My dad was a lawyer and I thought it would pique my interest. It didn't. I really was more like my mother. It was my brother, Herman, whom we called Harry, who was more like my father.

In fact, my brother and I are 180 degrees opposite each other. Like Dad, my brother is a Republican, whereas I'm a liberal. He's a radiologist and has money; I'm in public health and I don't have money. Part of that is because Harold followed my Dad's example. Dad was close to the belt when it came to finance. He and my mother would often go up to the Dairy Queen in Drayton to get an ice cream cone. I remember one time when Dad had a brand new Cadillac and they went up to the Dairy Queen and he found out the price had gone from 10 to 15 cents. He refused to pay it. He was so mad, he skidded his tires getting out of the parking lot.

On the other hand, he did better at finance than I did—both he and my brother. Harry and I have always liked each other, even though he saw things a little differently than I did. But he never saw the world like I did. I saw people in their personal situations. In veterinary medicine when you do house calls you get to know what people do, how much money they've got, whether they've got any intelligence. I think all doctors should probably go back to house calls.

When I was about to graduate, I interviewed for a job in a small animal veterinary practice in Topeka, Kan. My wife and I went down there with our daughter. They set us up in a motel and brought us over to their house and treated us to a cocktail. Well, we weren't exactly the cocktail set. I was lucky if I got a little time on Friday to go out and have a beer. I got a little drunk that night and maybe too garrulous.

I didn't get that job, but I was more interested in large animals, anyway. I did get hired, finally, by a veterinarian in Valley City, N.D. I borrowed a truck from the farm and we loaded all our earthly possessions into it. My wife drove the car down and I drove the truck. She was big and pregnant and on September 10, 1956 we were greeted by the prettiest girl you'd ever want to see. It was Barbara Lynn Eelkema and they said in the hospital she was the prettiest baby since Peggy Lee who had been born there.

So we ended up with two kids in Valley City. We had trouble finding a spot to live and finally settled on a small cottage. You could actually sit on the couch and tune the TV with your toes. We paid $75 a month and we rented out the basement for $50 a month to some college kids from Valley City. I saved money during that year. It was the first time I had a salary and a job.

The vet I went into practice with in Valley City, was only 40 years old. He was a chain-smoker and probably a round peg in a square hole. It amazed me how much time he spent kicking animals. A dog would come in and if he didn't do the right thing, this guy would kick him. And I thought that wasn't an appropriate thing for a vet to do. He should like animals. But he was a mean son-of-a-bitch and he was only 40. His wife was a little dizzy, so he put her on steroids which didn't make her any better. It was kind of a dysfunctional family. He died of a heart attack at 42. He was angry, a heavy smoker, hypertensive and he was not happy.

During those first two weeks, when my partner took off on his vacation and I became an instant horse expert, I also did my first cat spay. But I did it after I put the cat under with ether. Well, the cat died. I figured, well, I'll never get another cat to spay. But as it happened, they just brought them in for miles around. I didn't have any problem after that. I knew better than to put them under to the point that they died. Anyway, somebody brought in a bunch of skunk kittens and they wanted me to de-scent them and I wasn't really too happy about it. But I knew how to do it from vet school. So I got a table and I went outside the clinic and I took a very sharp knife and forceps and I de-scented all of those kittens. And pretty soon I was known as "the skunk de-scenter." And they'd bring 'em in from 100 miles away. I didn't really think people should have skunks as pets, but it was very popular at the time and so I had to vaccinate all of them.

Mostly the practice was in large animals. When you are in that kind of medicine you have to get up early in the morning and work late at night. A farmer would get into his barn about dawn and that's when he'd start seeing a sick cow. So that's when you'd get a call. During the day I'd go out and golf and enjoy life—or drool over the new Chevys. Then I'd get home and want to have supper and enjoy my family. Generally, about 8 p.m., I'd get a call.

Down on the Sheyenne River there was a group of Norwegian farmers who had never lost their brogue. One evening I got a typical call from one of them. He said, "Yah, the cow is calving. Can you come out?" I asked him how long the cow had been calving and he said since 8 o'clock that morning. I asked him why he didn't call me right then. "Oh," he said, "the local veterinarian is down the road. I had to try him first."

I thought, oh boy. I asked him if the cow was in the barn, but it was still out in the pasture. I told him to get the cow in the barn and I'd be out in about an hour. So I went over to the Highliner Café and had a cup of coffee and then I went out to his farm, about 20 miles south. I got there and he said, "Oh, I didn't think you'd be coming so soon." So then we had to waste an hour putting the cow into the barn.

When we did that he looked at me and said, "Oh, I don't know if I want you to work on my cow or not." I asked him why not. "Well," he said, "you don't look old enough to graduate yet."

That was pretty much the story of my veterinarian practice. I'd get these calls in the middle of night. I'd get so mad as I started out I thought I would charge the guy a big amount of money. At that time $100 was a lot of money. I'd go over to the Highliner Cafe and get some coffee and get in the car and the moon would be out. And I'd be thinking, well, maybe 50 bucks. And I'd get on the farm and there would be some kids there, barefoot kids, and the family didn't look like they had a lot of money. And pretty soon I was losing money. I came home one time and the TV wasn't working and I called for a repairman. He came over and charged me a huge price just for coming over. And he said, "Well, you know, I had to put gas in the car." He only had to come two blocks. And I thought, I don't know why I'm not charging for gas when I'm traveling all over the country.

But many of the farmers I dealt with didn't have a lot of money. One farmer, a Dutchman, had never seen a Dutch vet. He had a bunch of ruptured hogs. He wasn't sure if anyone could fix them. I went down there and fixed them. It wasn't any problem. He had one big ruptured boar and he said if it lived, he would butcher it in the fall and bring me half of it. And he did, all cut up and frozen. I didn't get any more than that. No cash was transferred.

That whole Sheyenne River Valley was made up of Norwegians and Hollanders. There were some Dutchmen from Friesland, which is where my family came from. But there were some from Gronigen, a province that borders Friesland to the north. When they found out I was from Friesland they didn't want to call me anymore. There was that kind of hatred between the two provinces.

I did make some money that year, but none of it was easy. I did a lot of service work. When you're the junior partner you get a lot of that stuff thrown at you—a lot of castrating, dehorning and de-worming.

There was a vet named Rossburg down in Castleton, N.D., a little bit out of our territory. But he had broken his leg and hadn't done a lot of his service work. He called me and said he had 200 bulls to castrate. And I said, "Fine, I'll do that." I went up there on a Saturday and found 200, 18-month-old Angus bulls with balls as big as my fist. Being young and dumb, I had them all put into a Quonset hut.

I had one farmer take hold of the nose end and another farmer would lift up the tail. I'd cut out one ball from one side, and then go around and get the other side. I cut off and tossed about 400 balls that day in a very, very warm Quonset hut that was running over 100 degrees. I only charged a dollar a ball. And I decided then and there that I wasn't going to be able to do that for the rest of my life. I decided that if I got out of that hut alive I would put in my application for medical school. I did, and so I did.

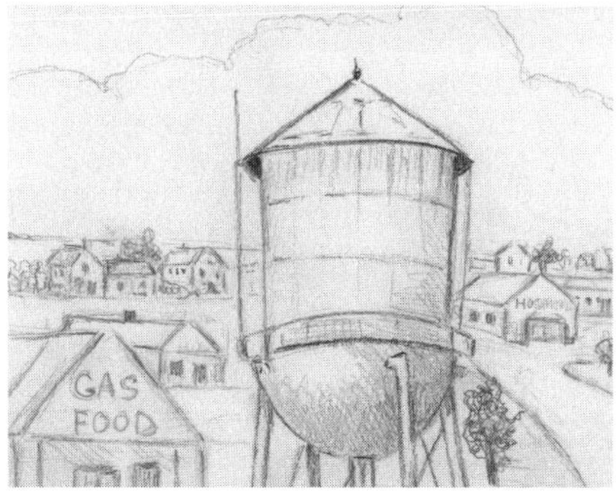

10

Ice on the River

JUNE 8, 2000, ANIAK, ALASKA

DARYL BJELDE IS a big guy. He is probably about an inch taller than I am and he probably has about 50 pounds on me. But I don't think he has changed much since he entered our physician assistant program back in 1977. He says that after he graduated he married a Sioux Indian down in South Dakota and she ran away with an orthopedic surgeon in Rapid City, S.D. He was never happy with that. But he is certainly doing a yeoman job in Aniak and he plans on going up to another spot nearby in September and starting another sub-regional clinic.

Aniak is as good a place as any to be called the middle of nowhere. There are no roads into or out of here. You either get there by booking a ride on a special 737 out of Anchorage that is fitted out to haul supplies, or you arrive by boat, float plane or snow machine. Someone said the word Aniak means "where it comes out," referring to the spot where the Aniak river flows into the Kuskokwim. The town of Aniak lies right at that junction. The closest big town is Bethel, about 100 miles southwest of here where the Kuskokwim flows into the Bering Sea.

Anchorage lies more than 300 miles to the east. We took that 737 and crossed over snow- covered mountain peaks that were just unbelievably beautiful. It was sunny and there was no wind. It was one of those unusual days in western Alaska that, believe it or not, was around 32 degrees. Last week it got down to minus 40. They get about five feet of snow up here every year, on average. We saw some mushers go by with their dogs. Daryl owns a couple of dogs, both of them are Siberian huskies. He lives alone in a house very close to his clinic. He said sometimes it is too close.

The village of Aniak is surrounded on three sides by dikes and the dike is probably 20 feet tall, at least. Usually, every spring during ice break-up, the water raises high enough to where it is pushing ice chunks over the top of the dike. On the back side, if the ice stops further down the river then the river water will start backing up. Daryl has been here five years and only once did the water back up so much that it reached the pad of the clinic. But the clinic didn't get wet. When they built it, they raised the level of the land around it to a spot where they figured the river would never get to.

Daryl works as a physician assistant for the Yukon Kuskokwim Health Corporation. As we arrived he told us that his president, his collaborating physician and two other doctors were going to leave early this morning from Bethel and travel up here on snow machines. They figured they would be here about noon. But their trip fell through. Before they make a trip like that they first go up in a float plane and they mark their trail. They did that last weekend. Right now the trail is pretty well marked, but there are areas where you have to drive on the river and they are saying there are open holes. The river has been so warm the ice on it is not solid.

Daryl has been up here since 1993. He was raised on a farm in Crystal, N.D., so he was already familiar with small-town needs. He came to our program as a graduate of the Bismarck Hospital Nursing School. For about 15 years after graduating he held several physician assistant jobs and even worked for a brief time in northern Alaska. A recruiter with the state's public health service in Anchorage contacted him and within four weeks he was flying into Bethel.

Initially he worked for a year in the emergency room of the Bethel hospital where he became friends with hospital administrators and the CEO of the corporation. They introduced him to the new idea of sub-regional clinics they were setting up out in the small towns and villages. Daryl advised them on the kinds of things they would need for an outpost clinic.

Each one of the villages in a sub-region—such as Aniak—receive money from the federal government to provide things for their people, including medical care. Private corporations were formed to assist villages and each signs a contract for the provision of medical care—such as running a hospital and setting up and running village clinics. The federal funds go directly to the corporation. Each clinic is responsible for a fairly large chunk of turf containing small, scattered villages.

Daryl's sub-region clinic in Aniak is responsible for the larger villages of Upper Kalskag, Unalakleet, Red Devil and Lime with populations in the hundreds, and smaller communities in between, the smallest with just 47 residents. There are 14 villages in all, across an area roughly the size of North Dakota.

"I have been to all of our villages at least once if not several times," he said. "We try to get out to the villages two or three times a year. Prior to the PAs moving up here, the doctors from Bethel would spend one hour a day and they would have certain villages that they were assigned to and they would call them on the telephone. Prior to that they would call them on the VHF radio and they would talk with them regarding cases that they have seen."

There are no physicians in the Aniak clinic, just two PAs, including Daryl and his PA colleague, Mike, and three community health practitioners.

These are local people who are essentially an assistant to the physician assistant. They go through a formal training program led by Daryl, learning to take vital signs, do blood pressure checks and how to treat common illnesses. One phase of the training covers long-term chronic care for diabetes and hypertension.

To supplement that, a doctor comes in two days a month. Daryl's collaborating physician comes up every other month and spends about three days doing chart review and any minor surgical or urgent care cases. Each of the villages has its own small drug formulary for medications which are dispensed after consulting with a physician. Any shortfalls are brought in by airplane.

Even the smallest of villages has some type of gravel or graded runway. "But not all of the villages have runway lights," says Daryl, "so you are very limited as to the hours which you can fly into these villages."

The clinic's maintenance man, a native named Archie, is also their vehicle driver. When a patient comes in by airplane from one of the villages, the pilot will call and let Daryl know what time they will be on the ground. Archie then drives the van to the runway and picks them up.

Flying, I learned, is a way of life up here.

"I didn't like to fly until I got here," says Daryl, "but, you know, there are no roads. There have been periods of three to five days or so where there has been fog or blowing snow or blowing weather. One thing I learned very fast here, if the planes aren't flying, you are not going anywhere. There have been times when the weather has been nice here and we have taken off to try to get to a village and the weather goes down. The plane just turns around and comes right back again."

In that case, I asked, what happens if someone comes in who is having a baby.

"They make it mandatory," said Daryl, "that with OB cases they must leave their village at 36 weeks gestation and either go to Anchorage or Bethel until they have their baby. There are too many chances of major complications with untrained people doing the deliveries. There are a lot of midwives out there who are not formally trained. So far, we have delivered about seven babies at the clinic. What happens is they fly out of their village and they get this far and it either storms or the weather goes down. No planes are flying and they are in labor. Or they will go into labor while they are coming in and then they show up on our door and there we are, delivering babies."

The sub-regional system that Daryl is part of has vastly improved the ability of people in the really remote villages to get to a hospital—and even to get back home. Daryl's overhaul of the emergency responder system was a key factor in that improvement.

"Just before we moved up here we had a volunteer fire department that was also our emergency responder," he said. "They would pick people up on a stretcher, load it onto the back of a tractor or snow machine and transport them to the clinic. At that time they would be seen by the community health practitioners who would call the physicians in Bethel. The doctor would tell them what to do or how to stabilize a fracture or what have you. The patient would then have to wait for the next plane that was regularly scheduled to come out to that village.

"Now, with sub-regional clinics like the one here in Aniak, we are kind of a hub that covers five different private flight companies that have regularly scheduled trips to deliver supplies to each of the villages in our sub-region. They probably have four planes a day landing at these villages. What they do now is take patients discharged from the hospital back out to the villages along with their usual supplies like groceries, food, fresh fruits and vegetables and what have you. They come this far to Aniak and from here that patient and those supplies are transferred to the plane of another company and flown out to the villages. That is how groceries and medical supplies and even patients get to their small villages. And when they get out there, if someone is sick who needs to be brought back in, then they put them in that cargo plane and bring them back this far.

"In the meantime, we took our volunteer fire department and we trained them into a licensed ambulance service that is strictly volunteer. We have them trained all the way up to EMT 3. But it took a lot of work. Every Tuesday night we had meetings and would do lectures for one hour with the volunteers and then we had to get the state to agree to send trainers in to get their EMT training certificates. Now they are getting so good that maybe once a month we will give them a class on, say, hypothermia or some type of case we have had recently. Last Tuesday night, for example, we talked about respiratory arrest in a pediatric case. When I first started we had a two-month-old with respiratory arrest, but we found out that our respirators didn't work. The baby almost died on us but Mike and I got her intubated.

"We have even trained ten high school kids and got their parents okay for them to carry beepers. After school hours and on weekends they carry the beepers and, if we need the ambulance for something, they respond. We will also take them out of school if we get a bad emergency where we need their assistance. That was going so well that some people complained. There was a person who called for the ambulance when he couldn't move because of back pain. He said ten people showed up in his bedroom and he was laying there in his underwear. Okay. So we had to say, 'Well, maybe only two people should go into the house, the rest of you stay out.'"

Daryl said that the life expectancy here used to be 60, just because of the hard living and lack of exposure to medical care. But now, the life expectancy is approaching what it is in the lower 48 states. "As non-natives come in, the natives are switching their usual food habits," he said. "They are becoming more westernized and we are starting to see more cardiac disease and diabetes, both Type I or juvenile diabetes, and Type II as the elders are living longer.

However, while Daryl obviously sees the benefit of pushing preventive medicine, the reality in the clinic is the steady need for acute care. The problem: he doesn't have enough trained medical people to handle anything but the urgent stuff.

One thing I didn't realize about Alaska that makes an efficient emergency response system so important: The leading cause of death in the state is injury—from snow machine accidents, boating accidents, drowning and so on.

"In my first year out here I had three bad head injuries from snow machine wrecks, so I started talking about injury prevention," he said. "We have injury prevention groups that go out and do firearm safety and they have a portable swimming pool and they take it out and do swimming lessons to some of the villages and get the kids then to learn how to swim. We are now pushing snow machine helmets pretty heavily. I have actually seen three people who I thought would never, never, never wear a helmet and they were wearing them. I thought, all right, maybe we are getting somewhere. One of them just happened to be the mayor of Upper Scalskag and I thought, 'Yeah, you go.'"

While travel by snow machine up here is essential, Daryl said he has learned to be extremely careful, not just in driving his sled but in knowing when to go out and when to stay home.

"I never go out on the river until I have heard that Sunny Cameroft has gone out. He is about 60 and he goes out on his snow machine and fur traps and stuff like that. If I hear Sunny has been out then I know the trail is marked and it's safe. Last winter we had one elderly guy who went out and didn't come home. It took us five days to find the poor guy. He'd gotten disorientated in a storm and crawled under a great big old pine tree and that is where they found him. Then, a month ago two people were reported missing down by Bethel and it was snowing heavily, a white-out situation. They had to wait two days to go out and search for them and they found one of the guys frozen to death not too far away from the snow machine. But they never found the second person. They figure this summer, when the snow melts, they will find his body."

Daryl makes it a point of emphasizing that safety need to all newcomers to the area. "I try to keep them from taking off on their own, because you can actually get into some conditions where the weather looks good here but after you have been out a half an hour you get into a white-out situation. We always tell them just to stop their machine, hunker down and wait. You never leave here without at least three days of water and food, because you never know when the weather is going to get rough and you are going to have to find a big fallen tree to crawl under and light a fire and sit there and wait until the wind dies down."

That rule also applies to boating, he said.

"The first time I went out with a group of people, we went boating about 200 miles upriver and I had problems with the motor. I was supposed to be back to work the next morning. Well, we didn't get back here on time. That next afternoon we were drifting back down the river without a motor and who pulls up beside me but the state troopers in their boat. The first thing they said was, 'Uh, you have been reported as being lost, missing.'"

I asked Daryl why he had to teach kids how to swim. They live on a river. Don't they grow up knowing how to swim?

"Well, I was surprised that very few of them know how to swim," he said. "I couldn't figure out why. I mean they are surrounded by water but even in the middle of summer when the temperature reaches a balmy 60 degrees the water is still probably about 40 degrees.

"I had a buddy who is a native guy. We were out fishing and he just jumped into the water and swam and came back, nothing to it. So I jumped into the water and almost died. I didn't realize it was so cold. I cramped up and just barely made it back to the boat and hung on while he pulled me to shore."

When Daryl graduated from our UND program, the idea of physician assistants and nurse practitioners was still very new. Not only were physicians wary of working with PAs and NPs but so were prospective patients.

"When I first came here and they had started the sub-regional clinics, all the villages said they wanted a physician, nothing less. I felt my background as a nurse carried more weight than being a nurse practitioner or a PA because nurses were very accepted. It took me probably six months for people to recognize what a Physician's Assistant can do. At first it was one or two patients from a village who came here. They were seen and they must have gotten good care because they went back to the village and the word mushroomed. Recently they had a survey to see if they still wanted physicians and their comment was 'no.' If you can put competent PAs in the sub-regional clinics, that is all we need because they can do anything the doctor can do."

Because of his confidence and strong personality, Daryl was able to convince the administrators back in Bethel as well.

"I think I was their first exposure to really a strong PA with a nursing background. When I first came up here, they had one health aide who had trained as a PA. I took a look at what type of things they were not allowing her to do. They were things that I was repeatedly doing prior to coming up here. I talked to several administrators in Bethel and explained to them what a PA can do. And they said, 'Say, you know, we really didn't know what to do with PAs.'"

The way Daryl sees it, a PA with prior nursing experience has an easier time of it than a PA who has never been a nurse.

"I am very glad I went and took the nursing first, especially if you are going to be working out in a rural area. Because you're going to need to start a patient on IV fluids or you're going to have times when you need to draw blood, or you'll have an emergency where you need to intubate somebody. From my nursing training, I've done many, many IVs and mixed medications and so forth. Now when Mike first started here without that nursing training, as far as starting IVs he had not the slightest idea of what to use. He is still reluctant to mix medications because he doesn't know what to mix them with."

Of course, being able to do many of the things a doctor can do, Daryl is very aware of his limitations.

"The thing that I like about the PA movement is you are always under the auspices of a collaborating physician," he said. "The nurse practitioner way of looking at things is that they are independent. I think, though, that if you are collaborating with a physician you feel more free to pick up the phone and talk to them about cases that are bugging you."

About three or four times a year, Daryl makes it a point to fly to Anchorage to get back into civilization.

"I'll spend three or four days in Anchorage where they have movie theaters and shopping. The excitement is going to the mall and just sitting there watching all the people come and go and you think, 'My God, where are all those people going?' Out here if you are driving along and you run into another person, you stop and visit with them because on the trail, you can be out there for hours and never see another person you know."

Soon, I was flying back to Anchorage myself and marveling

that someone could leave all the comforts of modern life behind. I enjoyed our visit and I give Daryl a lot of credit for what he's achieved. He has a lot of enthusiasm for what he is doing and he seems to be very happy with it.

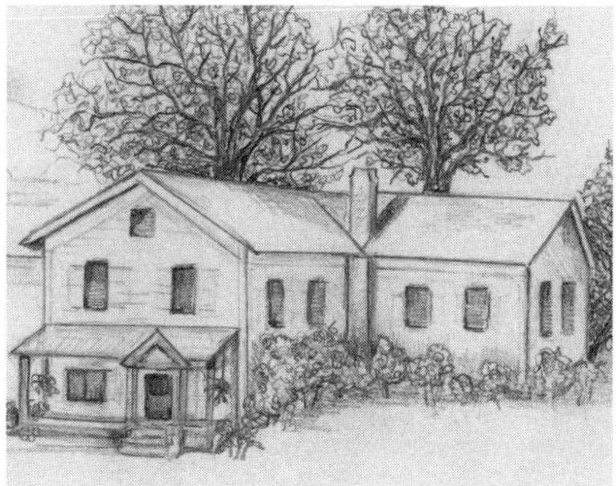

11

The Doctor and the Medicine Man

When I started medical school at the University of North Dakota in Grand Forks, I promised the dean—Ted Harwood—that I wouldn't have any more kids. At the same time we were incubating Katie. I thought that maybe when you were nursing one kid it would prevent another. Not so. Katie came 18 months after Barb, in 1958. I was pretty excited. I got a 100 on my biochemistry exam the day before she was born and a zero the day after she was born. All of a sudden I'm the proud father of three girls. I thought it was pretty nice.

UND had a two-year medical school at the time. About 15 years later I would play a role in the movement that led to the state's granting the school four-year, degree-conferring status. In the meantime, as a student, I think I did okay. I got the highest grade in biochemistry, having been well-steeped in that from veterinary school at the University of Minnesota. And I won the physiology award.

A curious side note about the culture of those times. I bet up to 80 percent of my classmates smoked. Everybody smoked then.

When he was 92, my uncle said the only reason he lived that long was because he quit smoking in 1950 when they came out with a scare. I used to go to class in medical school and smoke cigars in the front row. The guy that was giving the lecture had a cigarette hanging out of his mouth and was proud of it. That was physiology. Everyone smoked and the room was just blue.

All through medical school I practiced veterinary medicine on the side. I also helped with the school's animal lab. They had a terribly dirty animal reservoir and they took in a lot of dogs that had distemper. At the same time, they had research physiologists using the blood of those dogs in their blood-flow studies. I set up quarantine and immunization protocols to treat the animals before they were worked on from a research standpoint. I felt pretty good about being able to help them on that.

I sort of became known in the veterinary world of Grand Forks, to the point that when a wealthy woman died and left a pile of money to the Humane Society, they built a clinic and asked me to cover it as a vet. I had a vet technician covering it during day and he'd save animals for me to look at in the evenings. Meanwhile, on weekends I'd go out to nearby farms and test for TB and Bangs. I got money any way I could get it.

I made enough to cover the $1800 down payment on a brand-new house, 1,100 square feet, in a new area in south Grand Forks. The house cost $13,200 and I got $200 off for putting in the berm and the grass. At the age of 26 I'd bought my first home and I felt pretty good about that.

After two years at UND, we all had to find another medical school for the clinical training required to complete our M.D. degree. I applied to, and was accepted by, the University of Washington in Seattle. Ted Harwood didn't want me to go there because Washington had sent him a letter that said no one who was not in the upper third of the class need apply. He resented that, and a lot of my classmates went to Minnesota. But I looked at the average mean temperature in Washington and it seemed like pretty good country for me. So I left Grand Forks, if not on a high note, at least a very memorable one.

The speaker they brought in to give our commencement address was an honors graduate of the University of Iowa medical school named Dr. Vilhjalmur Stephenson. He was about 80 years old and had been raised from Icelandic stock in Mountain, N.D. He was a well-known arctic explorer, which must be why they invited him. But when he got up to give his speech, he said, "I have been waiting more than 50 years to tell this story."

Turns out he'd been a student at the University of North Dakota those 50 or so years ago and he'd gotten himself into some trouble. He got hold of the carriage belonging to UND's president and he parked it in front of a whorehouse. The president got so mad that he expelled him. The way he told the story was so funny. I mean they were so embarrassed at UND about the whole thing. But he was a great guy and I remember one of the last things he said: "They brought me back here, but they should have never trusted me."

Unfortunately when I transferred to Washington I went in the hole financially—mainly because I couldn't do any part-time work. I had to be at the clinic pretty much around the clock in those final two years.

We packed all of our furniture into a little trailer and the five of us headed west. That year, 1959, was kind of a depressed time in Seattle. Even though houses rented for $90 a month it was still too much for me. We finally got into a city housing project called Holly Park. It wasn't the greatest. I'd brought a jungle gym for the three kids and I left it outside like I did in North Dakota. But by the next morning, all of the hardware was stolen. And the tires to the kid's tricycles were gone. It was my first experience in city housing.

Later, when I came home in a white coat and everybody found out I was in med school, they brought back all the hardware. I became the local doctor for the unit. There were three buildings with six families living there. All were refugees from who knows what. I used to come home late at night, at 2 or 3 in the morning, and there would be five or six kids still be playing on the jungle gym. Every once in while a couple of kids would head on home, and a lady who was half dressed would shoo them away and say, "I'm not ready yet." She was obviously entertaining men.

My wife did some babysitting during the day for the mother of another family. She was supposed to have been home at 5 p.m. but she was out imbibing and didn't come home until 8 or 9. The husband of the family living next to us in our unit was a patient of mine in the VA hospital. He was in on a Section 8. For good reason. When he came home and found out his wife was pregnant—they already had three kids—he beat her up. We had a hole between our bathrooms—where we put the razor blades—and you could hear everything. His thesis was that he wanted to learn how to ski this winter, not pay the cost of another child. It was pretty sad.

The father in another family had been laid off from Boeing. He'd send his teen-aged kids to the market to steal sundries. He came home one time and found that a cop had caught his son. But all he did was whip him for getting caught. He got his comeuppance, though. He went out to Iowa to visit some relatives and when he got back there wasn't a stick of furniture left in his unit.

They had a central washing facility but you really didn't want to go down there. It seemed like there was a stabbing every night. It was not a good time, with people very often drunk and yelling at each other. It was my introduction to poverty after being a veterinarian and buying my own house. It was very difficult to take.

I did feel myself learning what you'd call "street smarts," something I didn't have before, because I had no need. One thing about Holly Park, everyone knew when the social worker was coming. All the men who were living with these women went out into hiding. The social worker was generally a buxom woman with a bag over her shoulders. She telegraphed everything and the word got around really quick.

The University of Washington prided itself on being the "Harvard of the West." They were just in the process of building a brick-and-mortar medical school when I was there. Most of our classes were in very old buildings and all of my clinical classes were scattered at three local hospitals.

During my time there we had three suicides. One of them was

a classmate. One was a neurologist who did himself in with phenobarbital and one was a dermatologist who used cyanide. My classmate was of Chinese descent and he'd been having trouble with English. It got him penalized in our obstetrics-gynecology classes. In order to bring his grades up he took summer school classes, but when he came back in the fall, he was broke. We had clinical conferences on Saturday and he parked his car in a no-parking zone. It got hauled away. He came home and told his wife it was gonna cost so much to get the car out. She really laid into him. He threw down his dinner plate and said, "Well, you won't have me to worry about anymore." He went out and drowned himself in 19 inches of water in the Japanese tea garden. That was really tragic.

The chairman of the obstetrics and gynecology department was an outright schizophrenic and he was a dangerous sort. He was a very sick guy. He would show up on the floor and insist that his medical students and residents review the patients with him, even though those students may not ever have seen those patients. They were so afraid of him they would present a patient's case with a conglomeration of the last two or three admissions. There wasn't anything truthful about it, very non-transparent.

I went down to talk to the dean. I said, "You know I came to medical school to help people and to increase their health. And I'm finding this is a pretty sick school with suicides in my class and faculty. I think you better examine yourself and what you're doing to these people. You're putting them on too high a standard and they can't live up to it. Get your psychiatric department involved and find out what the hell you're doing. You're creating more sickness than you're creating health."

Oddly, I didn't catch any hell for that, maybe because I was doing pretty well in school. He seemed like a nice guy. He was a Norwegian who came from Minnesota. But if I'd have been an average student, I would have been afraid to say any of that.

One of the best things that happened during the summer was being able to work with Dr. Rei Ravenholt, the epidemiologist in King County. He was looking into staphylococcus infections showing up in local hospitals. He wanted to find out if there was anything in the animal kingdom that might be spreading the staph.

We designed a study to visit the fish houses, poultry farms and pig slaughterhouses in the area. Because I was a veterinarian I'd go and talk to the local vet and tell him what we were doing. They were really cooperative. Anytime they had an animal that had an abscess in the ear, throat or liver they'd call me. I'd do a swab, and then I'd do a swab of the workers who had been working with that animal.

I also did it with fish in the fish market. People who caught rock cod—they have sharp spines on their backs—might puncture a finger. If that happened we drew blood and they got a shot of penicillin. We found that a germ living in the ocean was infecting the fish and then showing up in the blood of fishermen. It was *Erysipelothrix rhusopathiae*, the same virulent organism that causes erysipelas in hogs. It was just eye-opening for me to see that. We wrote an article in 1961 called "Staphylococcus in Meat-Animals and Meat Workers." One thing we weren't able to do was connect any animal organisms with the staph problems in the hospital.

But because of the project I became fast friends with Rei Ravenholt and his boss, Sandy Lehman, the county health officer. They really treated me well. When I wanted to start my preventive medicine residency, following my graduation from UW, they recommended me to the Center for Disease Control in Atlanta for training in the Epidemiological Intelligence Service (EIS).

The EIS is a unique two-year, post-graduate training program of service and on-the-job learning for health professionals interested in the practice of applied epidemiology. I started that in 1962 and chose to enter the Public Health Service Commissioned Corps, one of seven federal uniformed services that includes the Army, Navy, Marines and so forth. We were attached to the Coast Guard's public health services in Seattle. I did it because I felt guilty that I hadn't gone to the Korean Conflict. I'd been part of the Air National Guard unit in Duluth and they were going to send some of us to Korea. We drew straws to see who would go and who would stay home. One of the guys who drew the short straw got his toes and fingers frozen off over there. So I felt maybe I should go back into the service.

One of my first assignments was a six week stint at the Indian Health Service hospital at Fort Defiance on the Navajo reservation in eastern Arizona. It was not far from Window Rock, Ariz., which is the capital of the Navajo nation.

To get there, I took my first jet ride down to Salt Lake City, dressed in my fresh new uniform, a proud stripe-and-a-halfer. I stayed the night in Salt Lake, but I celebrated a little too much. I got on a DC-3 the next day and this time we didn't go over the mountains, we went through them. With the updrafts and downdrafts I thought I was going to die.

I remember hoping that I'd have a day or two to recover before I had to go to work. But when I got to Gallup, N.M., 30 miles east of Fort Defiance, I was met by a Native American who drove straight out to the hospital. A female orthopod welcomed me to the hospital's emergency room and said, "You're on." And she left me.

There were 15 to 20 kids in that ER, all with fevers, diarrhea and dehydration. The first thing to do was get fluids into them, but hooking a sick baby up to an IV line isn't as easy as doing it for an adult. I had to do surgical cut-downs on four or five of them to find a vein. Fortunately, as a vet, I knew how to do cut-downs and was quite practiced at it.

I remember our nurse, Mrs. Bailey kept putting wet towels on all of those kids. But so many of them had been brought in too late by their parents. What they did first when they saw their baby was sick was take it to the Navajo medicine man. He would wrap them up in blankets and put them in front of a charcoal fire and dance around them. It's the worst thing you can do to a baby who's dehydrated. By the time they got to the hospital they were so sallow, looking like little old ladies and little old men. It was very hard to get enough fluids into them to save them. I would say we didn't even save 50 to 60 percent of them. It was very, very sad.

The infant mortality rate there was bad. Some of the mothers let their young kids drink out of the watering trough for animals.

They soon got diarrhea and they'd come in and we had to hospitalize them. Often we got into a real battle with mothers who wanted to have the medicine man come in to treat the patient alongside the doctor. We said he can do anything he wants in the hospital but he can't build a fire. That was my introduction to pediatrics on a Navajo reservation. Without a doubt, that six-week experience made me think very seriously of a career in public health.

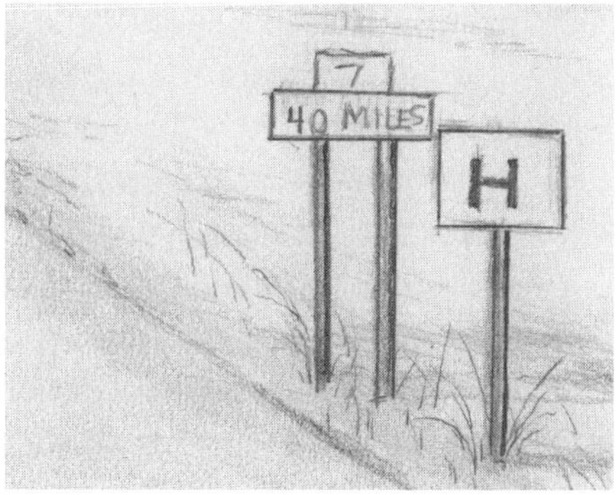

12

Doctor Territory

IF YOU READ much history you'll find that revolutions usually start out with a small, passionate group pushing for change, opposed by a much larger group—often including everybody else—pushing against it. Resisting an upheaval of the familiar and comfortable is only human nature. That is especially so if the norm seems to be in perfect working order and the revolutionaries appear as strident, unkempt ideologues with an agenda from the outer fringe. Even when they are reasonably kempt and only occasionally bombastic, agents-of-change usually are viewed as a threat.

With some notable exceptions, however, we find more often than not that the fringe is where progress is born. I'm not just talking about classic revolts that overthrow kings and dictators. But, from the laughable idea that illness is caused by invisible creatures called germs, to the uncivilized electrification of music that already seemed sublime without it, to the delusional ideas of an un-pedigreed inventor named Steve Jobs, the standard notion that something unbroken needed no fixing was always beside the point.

Revolutions aren't about tinkering or cosmetic renewal. In 1783, during the ceremony at Yorktown where Lord Cornwallis surrendered and effectively ended the American Revolution, the fifes and drums of the Continental Army mischievously played, "The world turned upside down."

The field of medicine has been stood on its head through the centuries by scientific breakthroughs and innovations that often were greeted with skepticism and dire warnings of disaster. Even the educated and much-respected Benjamin Rush, the leading physician of his day in late eighteenth-century America, saw nothing wrong with bleeding a patient to balance the body's so-called "humors." When our first president, George Washington, fell ill to an infection of the throat in 1799, his doctor bled him of between 40 and 80 per cent of his blood in a 24-hour period (sources differ on the precise amount, but none is lower than two quarts.) That a man who has lost that much blood while also battling an infection could live for 24 hours is a testament to Washington's strength. Of course, he soon died.

Modest as it may seem, our revolutionary training of health professionals who could extend the reach of a doctor into underserved areas of the country was viewed by many in the medical establishment as dangerous heresy. The great fear was that the sacred role of the physician was being undermined by incompetent practitioners of the latest do-gooder fad.

This opposition did not impact our training programs, which were funded through government and private sources. But it did make it very difficult for our graduates to go forth into areas of need and find cooperation and acceptance from their colleagues as legitimate medical professionals.

That resistance came from three areas. First were the prospective patients who, understandably, expected to be seen by a doctor, not someone called an assistant doctor nor a nurse practitioner, which must have sounded like a glorified nurse. Second and third were the general corps of nurses and doctors themselves who viewed PAs and NPs as everything from competitors to frauds to a mere nuisance. We had expected resistance from both of those groups, but had hoped that the physicians we selected as preceptors to our students—and who, in many cases, later became their supervising physician in the field after graduation—would be uniformly supportive. Most were, although many were not.

Part of our training program involved multiple inspection visits to a preceptor's office by myself, and either Mickey Knutson or Judy DeMers. We were looking for evidence of a good working relationship that included a student being mentored and not merely supervised, as well as a demonstrated respect for the role those students were hoping to fill.

Again, most of our preceptor relationships worked out well, especially once we were able to bring in students who had already formed a bond with a physician who was willing, even eager, to take on the mentoring role. Such was the case of one of our graduates, Jim Combs, a successful physician assistant whom I interviewed in Mesa, Ariz., in 1999.

He was a senior in the nursing program at UND in 1977 when he went to an appointment with his dentist in his hometown of Enderlin, N.D., during his spring break.

Remembering that visit, Jim told me the dentist "had, like, two hands and a foot in my mouth at the time and he always talked while he was working on you and all you could say was 'uh, uh, uh,' you know. And he asked me what I was going to do after graduation. I said, 'Well, I don't know but I want to follow a nurse practitioner around to see if that is what I want.' He said, 'Oh good, I know exactly who you are going to follow. You are going to go follow my son in Minneapolis and I will get it all set up and I will make sure you get a good experience.'

"I didn't even have a chance to say, yes, I would be interested. He said it was a done deal. So he set it up and I went ahead and followed his son, Allen Olson, who was a nurse practitioner and also a graduate of the UND program. At one point during the six weeks, Allen asked me what I wanted to do in the future. I said, well, I wanted to be a nurse practitioner but I knew I needed to have a couple of years' experience and, of course, my nursing license.

"He came in one day and he gave me a UND nurse practitioner pamphlet. I said I'd heard all about what an excellent program it was, but I still needed to have two years of experience. He said, 'Well, what if we wanted to get you in sooner? Would you go?' I said, 'Absolutely.' And he told me he had a doctor who was willing to take me on as a student. I went ahead and interviewed with him, Dr. Herbert Straight.

"He said, 'Why don't you go into the program now? I will take you on as a preceptor.' I was just flabbergasted. Here, my dream was coming true right there. So he went ahead and called Judy DeMers and got things set up for an interview. At the time, I did not have the two years' nursing experience and I hadn't completed my RN. When I went into the interview with Judy, I was very nervous. She invited me to sit down and she sat across from her desk and she started in and said, 'Hey, how is Allen Olson doing?' And we sat and talked and I thought, 'Well this is a good ice breaker. We sat and talked about Allen and then she said, 'Oh, by the way, you are in the program.'

"I was absolutely ecstatic. I remember I called home and said, 'Mom, Mom. I have a chance to get into the nurse practitioner program.' She said, 'Oh, that's nice. How are you going to pay for this?' Because I'd gone through four years of college with only a $1,500 school loan. They had paid the rest. I said, 'I don't know. I guess I'll go ahead and get a loan.' She said, "Oh, that is very good."

"So I got a $6,800 loan from my hometown banker, I finished taking my finals, got my RN and graduated from the UND program in 1978."

And, of course, the relationship between Jim and his preceptor worked out very well. It was a little rougher for some of our other graduates in the very early years. Sometimes the preceptorship went well, but in spite of a glowing recommendation, the student found he or she had to prove themselves all over again when they graduated and found a full-time job with another doctor.

That's sort of what happened with Dorothy Johnson, one of our first five students. When she entered our program in 1972 she already had been a nurse for 16 years and was then the assistant director of nursing at Mercy Hospital in Devils Lake, N.D. Her preceptor was a local doctor named Gilbertson. When Dorothy graduated in 1973 she went back to Devils Lake and worked in Dr. Gilbertson's practice along with several other doctors. But even working in the same practice as her mentor, things did not go smoothly right away.

"Back then, all the older doctors were very conservative," she told me when I interviewed her at her retirement home in Phoenix in 2000. "Some of them were kind of afraid to have someone step into their world. When I got there, one of the doctors didn't even want me to write a blood pressure on his charts. That was doctor territory as far as he was concerned. At first they still thought I was a nurse in the emergency room, you know, working as evening supervisor. But, that kind of wore down after a year or two and they got to trust me. I think it took about six months before I got my own appointment book, but some of us had to blaze the trail."

There were also doctors opposed to the program at first but who came around once they'd seen the usefulness and proficiency of our graduates. A perfect example of that was a Bismarck physician named Bob Tudor. He was one of the nine physicians on the Board of Councilors for the North Dakota Medical Association at the time I was drumming up support for the MEDEX Program.

I only needed to win the support of five councilors for their official blessing, but it was clear from the start that Dr. Tudor wasn't going to be one of them. He opposed the idea big time. He felt that PAs and NPs would be an intrusion into the practice of medicine. He would go to medical meetings and rail against using extenders, urging the board not to support MEDEX.

I was reminded of Dr. Tudor's story the day I visited with one of our graduates, Colleen Holzworth. Her preceptor had been none other than Bob Tudor and she could only sing his praises.

"He was almost like a father to me," Colleen told me when we met in May of 2000 in Grand Forks. "I mean, that man, if it wasn't for him, I think I would have had a few hurdles to jump. But he just sort of took care of everything."

What had changed his mind? Well, it turned out that Dr. Tudor had a niece who came into our training program. She'd been doing her training with a preceptor in Crookston, Minn. She wanted to finish out her preceptorship in Bismarck, where she was from, and she asked her Uncle Bob if he would help her. Blood being thicker than water, Dr. Tudor decided reluctantly that he would participate. Not long after he'd become Colleen's preceptor, he went out to the meetings of medical groups and told everyone that the program was the best thing since sliced bread.

Among our graduates in later years, we began to see that many young doctors had pretty much grown up with the idea of PAs and NPs. It was becoming an accepted part of the health care system.

The first physicians to come around to the new way of doing things went out and approached potential students without our prodding. They volunteered to be their preceptors if they went through a PA or NP program. They could see firsthand what kind of help they needed. I got a good feel for that when I spoke to Diane Cardwell in January of 2000 in Ames, Iowa.

Diane came into the program in 1989 with eight years of nursing experience. The doctor she was working with in her home town of Seneca, Kan., helped pay her way into our program. He served as her preceptor during training and after her graduation she became his physician assistant. When he eventually moved on from Seneca, Diane went with him and they started a family practice in an Ames clinic.

"When I first came to Iowa it was a little bit of a struggle for me. I practice today as a PA because it took me longer to get my NP license and I had to basically go to the Board of Nursing and explain to them exactly what I did. They were familiar with pediatric nurse practitioners and a little bit with geriatrics, but they just could not assimilate that into the role of a family nurse practitioner. They were kind of mesmerized when I described to them what I was used to doing and what I was doing as a PA and please give me my license as a nurse practitioner. They were kind of going, 'You really do all of this?'"

By then she had become used to ignorance as well as skepticism about her role. In Kansas, she recalled, "The nursing staff at the small community hospital there was very judgmental and very critical of my role. It just takes time. It was like if you don't make an issue out of it and if you just do what you do and you do it well, the care and the patients will speak for itself and that is exactly what has happened.

"But there are times when you need to make an issue of it. When I was first practicing here in Iowa, I was doing colonoscopies. We had a gynecologist and I would send him a referral for a treatment on an abnormal biopsy that had shown up during a colonoscopy I'd performed. And he would repeat the colonoscopy and charge the patient. I remember very distinctly going into his office and saying, 'You know, let's talk about this issue here. If you don't want my referrals then just say so. But I think it is a sin for a patient to be charged twice. If there is a clinical issue on something I have done wrong or misdiagnosed or was not done well, let's talk.' But he just was not going to trust a referral from a PA. So, I sent him no more referrals. I found someone else who would accept them.

"There have been times that patients have been scheduled with me and they would be a little appalled that they were not seeing a physician. And I would say, 'You know that is perfectly fine. We will get you in to see a physician and we will get you in fairly shortly.' I have always been very fortunate to have physicians that were very flexible. The majority of the time when that would happen the patient would say, 'Well, let's just see what you do and then, if I am not happy I will see the physician.' Typically that would be a non-issue. So, when I bring on new individuals here I will say to them, 'Let what you do speak for itself.' I think that probably leads to the most success."

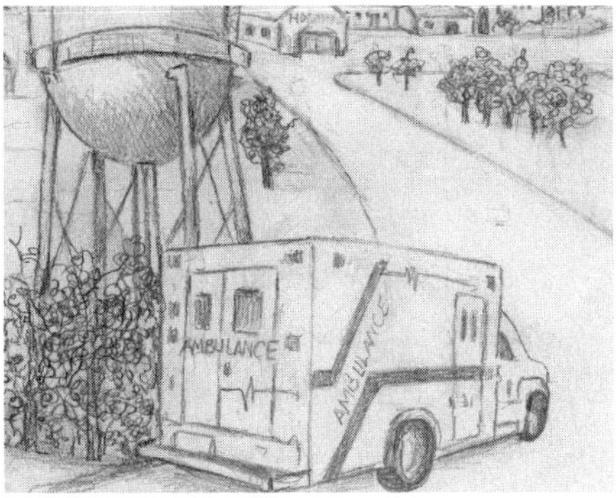

13

Fifteen Minutes of Fame

WHEN WE ARRIVED in Seattle in 1959, we had three little girls. By the time we left for my six-week training session in the EIS at the Centers for Disease Control in Atlanta in 1962, we had our fourth daughter, Jennifer Sarah, born March 16, 1961. At that point I was a typical, newly minted doctor with a successful career beckoning, but so far no cash in my pockets. I knew very well that my calling to the public health side of medicine was never going to make me rich, but I did long for the time when I could at least be breaking even again.

My income as a medical student at the University of Washington was negligible. I worked a deal with my brother to take my kids as tax deductions, which is allowable if you are paying the majority of their support. In exchange, he then advanced me so much a month. He didn't charge me any interest, but he kept a record of it and I paid him back in monthly installments. In the meantime, my dad—like a lot of farmers—was land-rich but very cash-shy. He came up with $5,000 but he made me pay it all back, which I did, every dime.

We sold all of our furniture in Washington, then packed everything else, plus four girls, into a '56 Chevy station wagon. En route to Atlanta in 1962 we drove across Mississippi. I remember very clearly two things about that crossing. One, it was the day William Faulkner died in Jackson, Miss. And second, we stopped at a laundromat to wash some clothes and there was a sign inside that said, "Whites only." My wife said, "Well we've got colored clothes too." We were pretty naïve.

In Atlanta we stayed at a hotel called Peachtree Manor, where the old Negro League Atlanta Crackers stayed. It was the only hotel that would allow blacks. We were integrated even if they weren't integrated in Atlanta. Surprisingly, during our EIS training we did a house survey in Atlanta and we noticed there wasn't any segregation in terms of housing. You could go to a block and find both blacks and whites. The schools, however, were strictly segregated.

The EIS was and remains a great organization. I got to know some pretty sharp doctors while I was there. There wasn't a dunderhead in the bunch. They all went out and got really great positions in academia or practice or in the National Institutes of Health. The big cheese at the time was the man who started the Epidemiological Intelligence Service, Alexander Langmuir. In that world he was an icon. He was also a perfectionist, the epidemiologist *par excellence.* I consider him a mentor.

There was one thing about the CDC that jarred me, though. We took our classes in a CDC auditorium where all the chairs had ashtrays. There were several smokers in our group, and nobody tried to stop them. It was still the going thing, two years before the surgeon general's report about the hazards of tobacco smoke.

Following our six-week course, I was recruited by Tom D. Y. Chin who headed up the EIS viral laboratory in Kansas City. He wanted to do a study of cold viruses at Father Flanagan's Boys Town in Omaha. Tom figured that since I had four young daughters, I must be Catholic and, therefore, would have an easy time getting access to Boys Town. Chin was an absolute genius when it came to virology, but he was wrong on this point. I wasn't a Catholic and, as we soon discovered, no one, not a Catholic, Protestant nor Jew was going to get access to Boys Town.

When we approached them, they were more interested in taking a donation than providing us any service. So we went into the Omaha Home for Boys, run by the Masons, who were very cooperative. Any time one of the boys came down with a cold I'd do a nasal swab and a throat swab and send it down to Chin in Kansas City. It turned out to be a fascinating study. We found so many different viruses it was almost unbelievable. At the time there was a faint hope that someone might be able to make some kind of vaccine for colds. But given the 150 to 200 separate viruses we found in Omaha—all of them causing the same symptoms—the idea of finding one vaccine that fits all became an impossible situation. If they ever do it, it will be a miracle.

I got quite a bit of experience working in Omaha. I was on the academic staff of the University of Nebraska and the medical staff of Creighton University where I'd lecture on epidemiology. I investigated a lot of food-borne type illnesses and published articles about them.

I also did a study of death certificates, covering every five years from 1880 to 1960. The idea was to compare the number of deaths across the years from things like childhood diseases, accidents and suicides. The one thing I learned was that death certificates back then were basically inaccurate.

When a patient died it depended on how sophisticated the doctor was when he signed off on the death certificate. If they didn't do a post-mortem exam, it was kind of a boilerplate thing. Most everybody who died suddenly, died of a heart attack. But you could tell if it was a suicide because most certificates cited the method. The doctor would write things like "putting head in oven," or "shotgun" or "hanging."

The only thing that changed regarding suicides was the method. The rate of suicide was the same over a period of 100 years: 11 suicides per 100,000. It impressed on me that even with suicide prevention programs, people will commit suicide at the same rate. I published this study in Nebraska medical journals.

While I was in Omaha I got called out to the Aksarben ("Nebraska" spelled backwards) racetrack to investigate an outbreak of equine influenza. I was then tasked to investigate racetracks across the Midwest and West. Because I was a vet, I could take a blood sample from a stable boy as well as the horse, to see if there was any antigenic similarity in horses and humans. I really hit a lot of tracks and became familiar with each track's veterinarian and doctor. Most of them weren't interested in influenza, but they did know a thing or two about horse-racing. Through them I learned how to handicap a horse race and became a life-long follower of "the ponies."

When I went to Omaha, our family came with me. We found an old colonial house a little past its prime and had just gotten settled in when I got a call from a pathologist at Methodist Hospital in Omaha. He said he had what looked like a case of polio in a young girl on their infectious disease ward.

One of the classic early symptoms of polio has to do with the trouble many victims experience maintaining a sitting position. They try to gain support by leaning back on their hands while bringing their knees slightly forward. When that happens, a sort of tripod shape is formed between the resting hands, the head, and the posterior. It's called the "tripod sign."

As it turned out, the pathologist who called me that day had survived a case of polio when he was a teenager. He knew all about the so-called tripod position and had seen it in this young girl. Yet he couldn't believe it was polio. Just 30 days earlier, Nebraska had completed a large scale vaccination for all three of the known polio virus serotypes.

Poliomyelitis is a virus that attacks the central nervous system. It withers muscles and can cause complete paralysis. In 1952 and 1953 huge outbreaks of polio swept the United States. Because it was a highly contagious disease, public health people warned kids to stay away from public swimming pools. When I first started training as a doctor, there were whole wards in American hospitals filled with people who couldn't breathe because their lung muscles had atrophied.

Those people, most of them children, were placed in what was called an "iron lung"—a tubular machine that worked the lungs in place of withered muscles. Researchers had long been working on a vaccine for what was often referred to as infantile paralysis. In 1954, Jonas Salk, a research virologist at the University of Pittsburgh, started unprecedented trials of a polio vaccine, injecting almost two million schoolchildren—known as Polio Pioneers—with inactive or dead strains of the virus. A year later, when the successful results of those trials were announced, newspaper headlines screamed, "Polio Routed!"

After Salk's initial triumph, a second polio vaccine was introduced by a Russian-born doctor, named Albert Sabin. Working as the head of pediatric research at the University of Cincinnati, Dr. Sabin developed an oral vaccine which proved in trials to be as effective at preventing polio as the Salk vaccine. The principle difference between the two was that Salk's vaccine used dead or inactive virus strains while Sabin's contained the live or attenuated virus. Also, in his research Dr. Sabin found that the polio virus incubated in the body's intestines, where it could move easily into the bloodstream. While the Salk vaccine immunized people against the effects of the polio virus, it didn't prevent it from that initial intestinal gestation in the intestines.

Sabin was so convinced that his vaccine was better that he tried to stop the use of the Salk vaccine. The National Institutes of Health eventually chose to promote Sabin's vaccine for use across the world. It was officially licensed for use in 1962. In the last 25 years, cases of poliomyelitis have fallen by 99 percent, according to the World Health Organization. In the late 1980s there were 350,000 cases worldwide, while today there are fewer than 1,500. Only four countries—Afghanistan, India, Nigeria and Pakistan—are still described by WHO as being at risk for polio.

Sabin, who was a medical doctor, and Salk, who was not, did not like each other. But because of that Omaha pathologist's phone call to me that day, the enmity between those two medical giants was something I was shortly to verify with firsthand experience.

From the Omaha pathologist I learned that the patient in question came from Valentine, a small Nebraska city near the border with South Dakota. The girl's family doctor had sent his patient down to Omaha where she would come to the attention of that pathologist. Initially, she had been referred to Omaha's Children's Hospital where surgeons opened the girl's spinal cord and found it to be normal. And yet she continued to have fever and her leg muscles continued to atrophy. She was eventually sent back to her home in Valentine.

When I examined her I took another specimen and sent it to CDC for analysis. The results were stunning. In her blood was found evidence of one of the three serotypes of polio—specifically, Type 3. But her poliovirus was tame. In the polio world there are wild and tame viruses. Wild is something circulating in the community, which is what you're trying to prevent. A tame virus is one that has been neutralized. It's what you're trying to accomplish with a vaccine.

So this girl showed evidence of a tame virus, meaning she had been vaccinated against polio and yet she still had developed atrophy of her legs. Sabin's live-virus vaccine, from which this girl's virus had clearly originated, was supposed to confer lifelong *immunity,* not *cause* the disease. What had happened to this girl from Valentine was supposed to be impossible.

Very soon after that we started getting reports around the state of similar incidences. In Atlanta, Dr. Langmuir was very cognizant of the political implications of these cases. News of them had the potential of undermining public confidence in vaccinations and destroying the whole program. He wanted all the data we could find and flooded Nebraska with several more EIS officers. We combed the medical records in every hospital in the state. We looked for anyone with lumbar punctures that had five cells and showed certain protein and sugar levels. Then we went back and reviewed the cases as they came in. We sometimes took samples and sent them down to CDC. Over a two-month period we found 11 cases of polio associated with atrophy of muscles. (We also caught some unrelated cases of the echo virus, encephalitis and other neurological diseases that had been missed.)

Shortly afterward, at an EIS conference in Atlanta, I presented a paper on our findings. Among those attending the presentation were Sabin, Salk and researchers associated with their programs. After I read my paper the session was opened up for discussion. I immediately sat down and listened to these two guys swear at each other like sailors. Belligerent? You never saw two people who hated each other as Salk and Sabin did. Salk thought his vaccine had done the job. Sabin said that wasn't enough. He said he developed the live virus which would give life-long immunity.

Sabin refused to admit that his vaccine had caused polio. He started nitpicking every one of the 11 cases we had discovered and presented. He argued fine points that had nothing to do with reality. He did get the committee to eliminate two of them. My thought was that whatever you wanted to call them, those two people in Nebraska with the atrophied legs didn't just pick up their pallets and walk because of Sabin's small victory.

Afterward, my paper was deemed by Dr. Langmuir as too volatile for publication. While we went back and investigated two more cases, CDC came up with a percentage chance of actually getting vaccine-associated polio. It was something like one in a million. I have no idea how they could come up with that or any such figure.

It was pretty exciting, however, to take part in that investigation and to play even a small role in such a contentious meeting of two men deemed heroes by almost everyone. My name was mentioned in a footnote in Mark Pendergrast's excellent book about the EIS, "Inside the Outbreaks." It was my 15 minutes of fame.

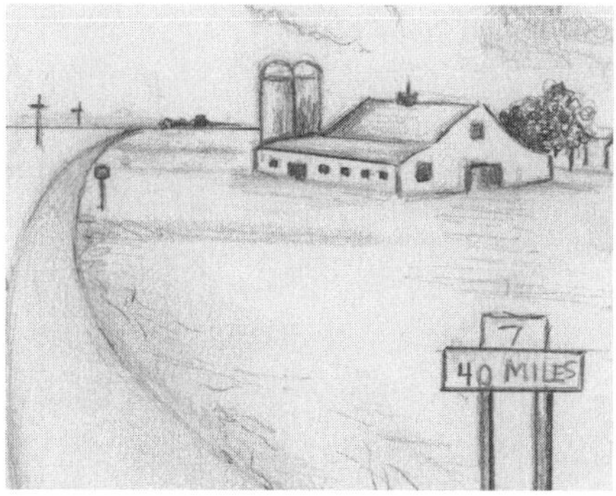

14

A Turn in the Road

IN MARCH OF 1964, while still in Omaha, we had our fifth daughter, Emily. I wanted to stay in the public health service but I had a lot of kids and really needed to make some money. I thought if I went into private practice I could support my family. Through a contact at UW, I was referred to a doctor in Snohomish, Wash., near Spokane and he hired me into his practice right away. I was entitled to one free move after I left the uniformed health services and I used it on our trek back to the state of Washington.

Once we got up there, though, just about everything went wrong. It was partly me and partly the doctor I'd signed on with. For one thing, we couldn't find a decent place to live. All we could find were two-bedroom houses, but with five girls it was tough. We stayed at the doctor's house for a while but he had a cat that scared the daylights out of the kids.

I soon found out that this doctor's practice was going to hell in a hand basket. Two of his partners had left him. Meanwhile, he was trying to buy the clinic and was borrowing 90-day notes just to pay my salary. There were also a lot of things about his idea of a doctor's role and just plain ethics that grated on me. One day when I was doing a routine exam on a young girl, he came in and whispered to me, "Don't tell anybody she's got small tonsils. We may have to take them out next week."

That was the straw that broke the camel's back. I quit the practice and we packed up the kids and went out to Sun Lake State Park, east of Spokane. We camped out there for three weeks. I didn't know what I was going to do with my life. I started listing things that were important, but I just couldn't decide. I'd gotten this far in life and things just didn't fit. I kept thinking that I must have been made from a different mold.

On the other hand, I did own a house back in Grand Forks. By the end of the year we were back in North Dakota, living temporarily with my parents at the farm in Drayton. While we were there, Dr. Ed Lyman of the Omaha-Douglas County Health Department dropped in and I remember Dad playing his mandolin during his visit. Ed tried to recruit me to come back to Omaha to be their epidemiologist. I sort of wanted to stay in North Dakota. Even though I didn't have a job, I figured I could probably get one. I stonewalled him. I really liked him and he liked me and maybe if I'd gone back there, things might have turned out a little bit different.

But you never know where your turn in the road is going to be. Sometimes you can't even put your finger on why you're making that turn in the first place. I certainly didn't have a goal anywhere near what eventually happened. I kind of went with my stomach, my gut feeling. I wanted to do something that made me feel satisfied and worthwhile. I knew that preventive medicine was my bag, I liked epidemiology and knew it fit in well with my vague ideas about the future.

Not long after Ed left, I was downtown, walking to the Grand Forks YMCA. A friend from the medical school, Dr. Wally Wasdahl, chief of pathology, saw me and gave me a ride. He wanted to know what I was up to and I told him I wasn't sure. He said Dean Harwood needed a doctor at the student health services, so I went over to see him. The dean said he didn't have a full-time salary for a doctor, but said I could teach physiology half time. And I said, "I'll take it."

I spent half of my time teaching nurses and medical students and the other half working at the health service. It was run by a nurse named Ruth Noren. She was the kind of person who, if she saw somebody who had appendicitis she'd go to the doctors and tell them, "I've got somebody who has appendicitis." Most of the other doctors would get really upset with her because she had diagnosed it which, supposedly, was their territory. But she was generally 99 percent right. She'd take blood tests and take a white count and, if it was up, she'd do an exam. She was perfect. She was my ideal of a mentor for a nurse practitioner or physician assistant, real world evidence that nurses could do more.

I was on call 24/7 for student health duty. I had to carry a beeper, and even though I was half time I'd have to go in and see patients who showed up at the emergency room of the hospital. I was really getting tired. I finally went to the Third District Medical Society in Grand Forks and said I needed some help. I asked them to campaign to the university to free up some money for doctors who could make calls at night. And they started lobbying the university to do that.

In the meantime I was back working with the animal quarters and trying to clean that up. But I soon realized that all of it was kind of a dead-end situation. It was not getting me anywhere.

I'd completed my two years of preventive medicine residency and all I needed was an academic year to finish my preventive medicine boards and get a Master in Public Health degree. I looked all over the country and the one that intrigued me most was Berkeley. I put in my application in and got accepted right away for a public health fellowship. UND freed up some money to help me out. I moved everybody out there in 1967 and rented a house in Walnut Creek about 20 miles east of Berkeley. This time there were six kids. We'd just had our first boy, Robert.

Most days I'd get up at 5 a.m. and take a bus into Berkeley. It was a two- to three-hour, round-trip commute. When not at

Berkeley, I worked in a local emergency room. It was a very exciting year and very stimulating. Some of my instructors had won a Nobel Prize. The free speech movement was underway, with all of the "flower children." Sproul Hall was just seething with advocates and agitators and people like Cesar Chavez and Bobby Seale would come in and talk. I ended up staffing the Haight-Ashbury medical clinic on Fridays.

The first week I was there I asked several people in the program if they wanted to go out for a beer, just to get acquainted. But public health types are very straight and no one was interested. Then I got to Dr. Bud Shutt, whom I didn't know at all. I asked him if he wanted to go out for a beer and he said, "Gimme five seconds to think about it." From that point on we were best friends.

My graduation was easily the best I have ever been to. It was at the football stadium and everybody had flowers. At one point, the chancellor said, "Will all Ph.D. candidates stand up?" And they stood and he said, "You now have got your Ph.D." Then he said, "Will all the master's candidates stand up." We did and he said, "You now have your master's degree." Then he went on to the baccalaureate and then he gave the commencement speech. And what I remember him saying was, "This is the generation that says, 'do your own thing.' All I say is, do it where you are at."

Without a doubt I knew that "at" for me was North Dakota. During my year in Berkeley, Dean Harwood had called and said he wanted to start a Department of Community Medicine. He wanted me to start it up. So in 1968 the eight of us went back to Grand Forks where I took over as chairman of a new department devoted to public health. My future was suddenly a lot less vague than it had been.

One of the first things I did as head of the department was to hire a veterinarian to take charge of the animal quarters and to make sure our research labs were clean and suitable for credible research. I also started teaching a course in public health, assigning medical students to various epidemiological studies. One of them, which we got published, studied the frequency of automobile accidents involving people who had been hospitalized at the state mental hospital in Jamestown. (One of the medical students who took part in the Jamestown study was Jim Brosseau, the doctor who would take over the Department of Community Medicine when I retired.)

We reviewed all the discharged patients from 1965, dividing them into psychotics, neurotics, personality disorders and chemical dependencies. We checked their driving record 15 years prior to being admitted and 10 years after they were discharged. We matched that with a control group established by age, sex and geographical location with the help of the Safety Responsibility Division of the state Department of Health. We looked to see if there had been any decrease in accidents among the hospitalized vs. the non-hospitalized. It proved to be a very exciting study.

There appeared not to be much of a treatment effect among the psycho-neurotics or the personality disorders. But there appeared to be some treatment effects among the psychotics and chemical dependencies. But the most interesting finding was that there were 55 single-car accidents among the hospitalized group and only two among the control group, all matched for gender and geographical location, and years of driving. So I went back and reviewed those 55 accidents and divided them up into suicidal ideation, suicide attempts, and suicide-homicide attempts. I found there was a definite increase in suicide ideation and suicide attempts among that single-car accident group.

I presented this data at a conference in Detroit. This was evidently the only way they could kill themselves and still be able to have their family collect on the insurance. It kind of fell on deaf ears. Under old English Common Law, anybody committing suicide loses their endowment and their inheritance. And that was incorporated into American law as well. There had to be a way to do it without letting anyone know they were committing suicide.

Another study I assigned focused on the attitudes and feelings of doctors who were practicing solo, or perhaps with one partner, in rural North Dakota. There were only about 250 to 300 doctors out there in what some have called "The Vast Lane" of North Dakota at that time. I sent students to small towns such as Hettinger,

Rugby, Dickinson, Gunnison, Carrington, Cooperstown and Rolla. We found that many doctors out there in the countryside were approaching retirement age and were looking, almost desperately, for associates to help with the workload. Some of them were able to attract associates but they'd end up giving them all the work and none of the pay. With that kind of inequality it wasn't surprising that a lot of people wanted no part of it.

Which is why, when I heard about Dick Smith's MEDEX Program I thought it would be such a perfect solution. By serendipity, as we were developing our MEDEX Program—and in regular contact with the Division of Health Manpower Research in the National Institutes of Health—we found ways to fund two other projects that have proved enormously successful.

As I've mentioned, the UND School of Medicine offered a two-year program and had been since its founding in 1905. There were a dozen other two-year schools like it around the country, but many of them, by 1971, were either closing or expanding into a full four-year, degree-granting program. With renewed interest in the medical profession, it was becoming difficult to find four-year schools that had the space to accept two-year grads as transfers. Dean Harwood and other deans before him had done well, placing their two-year grads in four-year programs at Harvard, Yale, Michigan, Minnesota and Washington. But the handwriting was on the wall: the day of the two-year medical school was coming to a close.

It left North Dakota with two choices: close or expand. Bean-counters in the state legislature favored closing the school to save money, oblivious to the need for homegrown doctors to serve their constituents. They were supported by many doctors in North Dakota's metropolitan areas who believed a four-year medical school could never survive. They argued that there was no city hospital in any of the state's small cities that could draw on enough patients for significant interaction with medical students. It was the reverse of the "Field of Dreams" theory for building a baseball park in the middle of an Iowa farm. "If you build it," grumbled many doctors, "they won't come."

During one of my trips to the NIH offices in Bethesda I told our MEDEX contract officer, Dr. Doug Fenderson, about the opposition to expanding the medical school in North Dakota. Remember, Fenderson was born and raised in the small North Dakota town of Streeter. He began telling me about a new federal program designed to alleviate the paucity of doctors in underserved areas. It was called AHEC, which stood for Area Health Education Centers, and was created to provide educational funding for worthwhile programs aimed at filling the doctor gap in a given area.

He thought AHEC was a potential solution to our problem. It was true that no one city in North Dakota had the population or the hospital facilities to serve as the teaching environment crucial to a medical school. But what if, instead of one large, centrally located hospital and medical school, we established a base in Grand Forks and created three other satellite campuses in the state's main population centers of Fargo, Bismarck and Minot.

Each of those campuses would become an AHEC location. Each could specialize in specific fields of medicine, and UND medical students could spend parts of their training in rotations at those various AHEC sites.

It solved the two main arguments against expansion in one breath. No one city could supply all the patients but split among the four corners of the state, each AHEC would serve a catchment area sizable enough for a unique training program for medical students. As for the cost of a four-year school being too high, the NIH would fund the AHECs.

My handball partner, Tom Clifford, the new president of UND, was a strong believer in a four-year medical school. He recruited me and several of my medical colleagues to join him in selling the AHEC idea across the state. While our campaign had its rough moments, we eventually convinced doctors and politicians that it could be done. In our 2003 book, "Good Medicine," Tom and I told the complete and engrossing story of "How wit and guile saved the School of Medicine at the University of North Dakota."

As if juggling the MEDEX Program and the medical school

expansion wasn't enough to keep me busy, a third ball was soon tossed into the air. It was tossed there by Doug Fenderson who noted that the Division of Health Manpower in the NIH was opening up a new division of Minority Health Manpower. The man Fenderson appointed to direct that division was a Native American dentist, Dr. George Bluespruce, who had been a classmate of mine at Berkeley.

Fenderson had already suggested that we consider developing a program to provide medical education to minorities. I loved the idea. I thought there should be a program on reservations for math and science, something that would get kids there prepared for college. Then I thought there also should be a college program that would not only combine tutorial and financial help, but also cultural support. I had seen many Native Americans come to campus for the first time. Because they were a minority, many of them became disenchanted and just plain lonely and would drop out and go back to the reservation. So we needed to provide cultural stimulation for them to stay in school. The sad fact was that there weren't many of their own people who had gone to college who could serve as a role model or a mentor. It's hard to break that cycle when you don't have any support from home to go to college. You need an awful lot of financial and emotional and peer support.

At any rate, we got the medical school to agree to take five Native American Indians into school. (At the time, the term "Native American" hadn't really caught on in many parts of the country. In North Dakota, where there are three reservations, the residents were still referred to as Indians.)

We also got the support from some of the Indians already on campus. The long and the short of it is that we got funded for a program we called INMED, for Indians into Medicine. And it has been a very successful program. Since 1973, the university has graduated 127 Native American physicians which is about 27 to 30 percent of all of the practicing Native American physicians. And I can say I was there right from the very beginning.

By the way, the only Native American graduate of UND?s School of Medicine at the time was Dr. Lionel DeMontigney who happened also to be my classmate. He became assistant surgeon general in the Indian Health Service and was instrumental in providing leadership to the get the INMED program going.

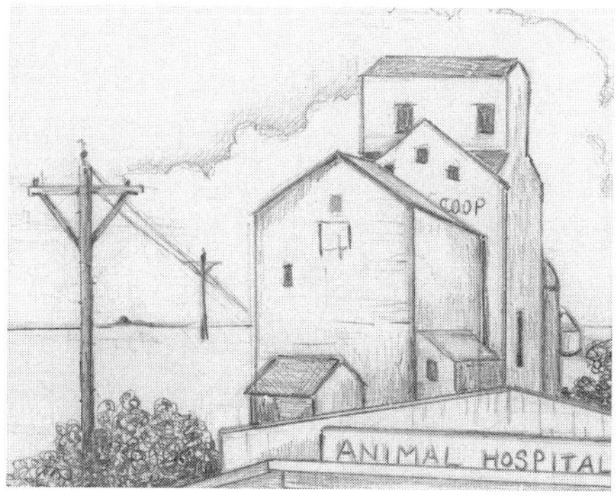

15

Staples of Medicine

NOT ALL OF the problems that developed with our preceptors in the early days of the program had to do with an unwillingness to cooperate. A couple of doctors who took on the mentoring role brought with them hidden personal issues that put our graduates in a difficult position. One of them actually put me in a very painful position, although, as it turns out, my own naiveté was the real root of the problem.

What I found reassuring, however, is that the graduates who had to deal with the human failings of their mentors rose to the occasion and performed admirably in the thick of things. I'll start with the situation Rick Gardiner found himself in after he completed our program.

Rick was a native of Montana who served in Vietnam as a corpsman during the 1960s. He was one of our first MEDEX students and I still remember his letter of application. He said he was somewhat of a rodeo rider and had fractured a few bones in the process. He said he once rode a bull by the name of Epsom Salts and he fell off and spent most of his life after that soaking in a solution of the same name.

After Rick graduated from UND he worked as a physician assistant in a small North Dakota town under the preceptorship of a young doctor who had been sent out by the National Health Service Corps. That's the federal agency that loans students money to help pay for medical school. In return, after students earn their M.D. degrees, they agree to spend a number of years in an underserved community, essentially paying off the loan.

This doctor, however, had two problems. One, he came from back East and was a raw, inexperienced city boy who was like a square peg in a round hole out in rural America. Secondly, he had a serious issue with alcohol.

"Big time," Rick told me. "It would get really bad. He was coming in to the clinic at 10 or 11 a.m. and leaving at 3. I was essentially on call every night because people in the community would see his car parked in front of the bar, so when their kid was sick they would call me and so I would come into the clinic and see their child. And in the morning he would come in and check the ER book to see what had gone on the night before, and he would never say a word. It was fine with him that I was showing up on his nights. It didn't bother him.

"What happened a lot is that people would just start coming to my house. There were some migrant workers jammed into a van up near Drayton, one time, and they got in a car wreck. The locals brought them all to my house on a Saturday, six of them, and they were laying on the carpet bleeding all over. I will never forget that. I had to call the ambulance to come to my house to take them to the hospital in Grand Forks."

Aside from the doctor's drinking, Rick said, the man still had a lot to learn about being a doctor.

"He would say, 'Rick, help me on this patient here. Here is the book, now I'm going to examine the patient. You read to me how to do the exam.' And this is right in front of the patient. I said, 'I don't know if that is a real good idea.' I would go into my office and read from the book. He would say, 'No, no, I want to do it this way.' And his patient's eyes would get this big around because

I would be standing there, reading from the book, while he was trying to do whatever exam it was. And you know, I just, I told him I am not going to do that anymore. Either get a stand and put your book on it so you can read it, because I am not holding and reading."

Eventually, said Rick, things came to a head. It happened one night during a blizzard when a pregnant woman and her husband came into the clinic. She was about to deliver, but the doctor was nowhere to be found.

"He went out of town," said Rick. "He claimed that we didn't have to stay in town. The father-to-be and I both told him, 'Yeah, we do. You can't go out in the blizzard. The roads are closed.' Well, a little bit later we couldn't find him. And this guy's wife was getting very close to delivering.

"I said, 'Well, you know, I have done a lot of deliveries in Vietnam, so we are okay. Don't panic here, because we will find him sooner or later.' We scrubbed the clinic down and then, just before she delivered, this frozen icicle comes through the door. He had driven out and couldn't see where the road went. There was a ramp going up to the Interstate and he had driven off it and sunk his car out of sight in the snow. A semi went by and he was standing on the roof of his four-wheel-drive waving the truck down. And the trucker brought him in and he was so cold he was shaking, so we did most of the delivery. He kind of just sat there and it was not long after that, that he kind of went off the deep end. He just couldn't handle it."

I have seen again and again that the abuse of alcohol and drugs is not limited to young people, especially in remote, rural areas. Even doctors, who should know better, fall into addictions. I remember, in particular, a doctor in Carrington, N.D., who was the preceptor for Bert Murphy, a 1976 graduate of our program. I spoke to Bert about her experience when I interviewed her in Jamestown, N.D., in May 2000.

She came to us as a practicing nurse with more than 20 years' experience. She'd married a rancher and had five children. I was most impressed during our talk with her great outlook on life. She loves what she is doing and she is a round peg in a round hole. At the time of our talk, Bert was working at the Jamestown State Hospital. But just after graduating from our program she had worked in Carrington with a doctor whom I'll call Dr. Rumboldt, who didn't treat her very well.

For one thing he didn't pay her more than $600 from the beginning to the end of each month for 15 years. "I would ask him for raise and he would say, 'Oh, that is all you are worth.' Yet very often he would push Bert into doing many procedures that she felt were beyond her scope.

"I did suturing and I even caught a couple of babies when he wasn't in there. I did rupture a few membranes and had to do a lot of suturing. I did almost everything. I mean, night and day I was on call." The reason Bert was continually covering this doctor's tail: he was addicted to pain-killers. Often he would simply disappear, but even so, Bert managed to keep him out of trouble.

"I would just tell the patients, I have to go get him, you know, or somebody has to go get him. But I would give them a choice. I would say, either we have to do this or you'll have to go somewhere else. They were usually willing to wait if it was an emergency."

Oddly, however, Bert, who has the patience of Job, still respected Dr. Rumboldt.

"Yeah, I respected him in a lot of ways for his ability to do what he did. You know, he came there as a young man. He knew all the people and they were good to him and he to them."

Mostly, Bert said, she felt she was in the learning mode and so she didn't complain. She felt it was a privilege to do what she did and she worked at it very hard. She said her professional satisfaction was her ability to do what she is doing.

Sometimes, though, she was treated by some of the other doctors in the same practice with raw hostility. But for all of his problems, said Bert, Dr. Rumboldt kept her under his wing and protected her from a lot of that petty obstructionism. I don't think that the young people coming out now recognize the terrible ostracism that our early students had to go through in order to accomplish what they accomplished. They really had to plow new ground. The rules and the laws and the activities had to be sort of moved along by feel. But most of them were steadfast and did a hell of a job.

I do know this: if Dr. Rumboldt hadn't had Bert, I dare say he would have lost his license. Bert covered his tail more than he will ever, ever know. He was such a lucky man. I just marvel at her capability and loyalty.

I also marvel at my own capacity for foolishness, a trait given its full head in an absurd moment in the mid-1970s when I was supposed to be judging the professionalism of one of our preceptors. It came about when Mickey and I flew to Idaho for a site visit with the preceptor working with Rick Perry, one of our early graduates.

After graduation, Rick took a job at a clinic in Lewiston, Idaho with a preceptor named Dr. Stipe. Mickey and I had just walked into the doctor's office when we were confronted with a crazy wall poster of an enlarged, inverted ear.

I asked Dr. Stipe what that was all about and he said that he performed ear stapling. He called it acustaple. In a way it sounded like acupuncture for the ear. He said he had identified certain parts of the ear which are linked to certain nerves in the brain that control appetite and smoking. He said he inserted a staple into the ear and, depending on whether he placed it horizontally or vertically, you could lose weight or quit smoking.

Well, we were mesmerized by the whole concept. Mickey wanted to quit smoking and I wanted to quit eating so much. So Dr. Stipe ended up anesthetizing our ears and inserting staples. I can't remember if they were horizontal or vertical, but he did put one in each ear. He said if you live more than 40 miles away, you probably needed it for both of your ears. Well, it was one of those things that sounded perfectly logical at the time.

No sooner had we been stapled than I met the nurse who worked with Dr. Stipe. She was extremely obese and, I noticed, she had a badly infected ear. I asked her what happened and she said she'd been stapled by Dr. Stipe so she could lose weight. It worked for a while, but then it got infected at about the time she was moving to a new house. I wondered later if it was more than 40 miles away. Because I noticed that only her one ear had been stapled.

Afterward, Dr. Stipe took us out to the airport in his new Cadillac. I was more than a little surprised to see him smoking a cigarette. I said, "Well, didn't you use your staples for yourself as far as smoking is concerned?" He said, yeah, he did and he still had his staples in his ears and he has cut his smoking in half.

We got on a small plane and we went up over the mountains. I can't remember what kind of plane it was but Mickey and I were in the back and all we did was laugh. We just couldn't believe that the two of us allowed him to put staples in our ears. I remembered a song that went, "My Mommy said not to put beans in my ears." I wondered if there was a song about staples.

Later on, when we got home, I knew I had to get those staples out. But I was very embarrassed about asking one of my colleagues to remove them. So I went to the warehouse at the Home of Economy where my wife worked, and she removed them with wire cutters and a pliers. Mickey forgot all about hers until she was taking a bath one night and started scrubbing her ears. All of a sudden the wash cloth got hooked into one of her staples and she yelled out bloody murder. Her husband, Larry, rushed in and said, "What's going on?" She said, "Well my washcloth got caught in my ear!"

The whole thing was kind of a bad experience but we got a lot laughs out of it. But the thing is, Mickey never quit smoking and the only weight I lost was the weight of those two staples.

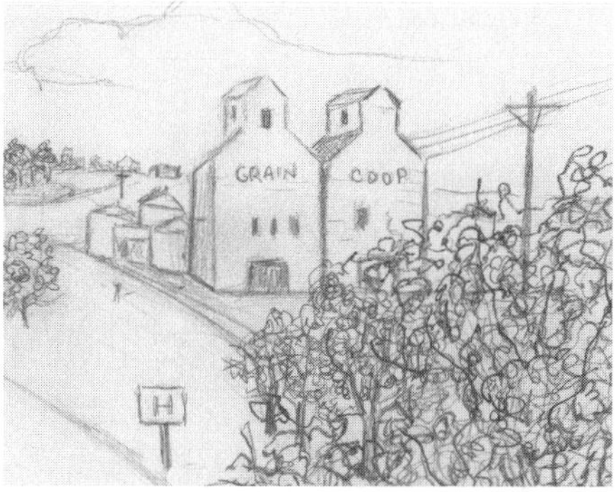

16

The Edge

WHILE I PROVED naïve about ear staples and could later laugh about being such a fool, I'm afraid my real blind spot was in failing to see the staples coming loose in my own life. While I'd been devoting all my energies to starting MEDEX, expanding the medical school and launching the INMED Program, I had taken my marriage for granted. As a result, my wife fell in love with another man.

When the divorce papers were delivered to me at work in 1972—demanding the house, the kids, my salary, the pension and everything—I was shocked. I had been away for so long trying to develop grants and contracts that I had neglected the life going on around me. Suddenly I needed to get an attorney to start defending myself. It was one of the hardest times of my life, just absolutely, totally depressing. I didn't know exactly what to do.

This all happened around Thanksgiving of that year. I took the kids to New York and we saw the Rockets, we saw "Jesus Christ Superstar," we saw "Forty Second Street." We did every kind of thing that there was to do. We took a boat around Manhattan and saw the Statue of Liberty. Basically, I tried to do things with the kids I should have done before. And I tried to forget about what was really going on.

Of course, it was impossible to forget that I had six kids and had to support them and keep the family going. To do that, I had to fight for custody of those kids.

The man my wife fell in love with turned out to be a person I hired to help in the MEDEX Program. They announced in front of the kids that they were going to take everyone out to Oregon to watch the sunset and live happily ever after. The kids were pretty much all teenagers by then and they didn't want any part of that.

The long and short of it is that I got a good attorney and we went through the divorce. I was able to salvage a little bit of money and keep most of the kids with me, and we got a reasonable divorce settlement. And although my ex-wife did go out to Oregon and did take a couple of kids with her, they came back almost right away. They wanted to stay with me.

I always like to think something positive comes from every negative. I think what that process did was to give me a lot of empathetic understanding and humility. I think I became a better person because of it. I went out to LaJolla, Calif., and worked with the psychotherapist, Carl Rogers. He helped put me on the right track. He gave me a positive frame of mind and got me thinking about starting life anew and getting on with the world and not ruminating over past losses.

Sometime after the divorce was settled, I had a routine meeting with my lawyer. I said something about being lonely and he said, "Why don't you take Ginny out?"

I said, "Ginny who?" And he said, "My ex-wife."

I would soon find out that my lawyer had lost his four kids in a divorce settlement for much the same reason that my ex-wife had lost hers. He'd been playing around and got caught. He'd told his girlfriend that he was cheating on his wife because she was a lush.

It wasn't the best recommendation for a prospective relationship but, as I said, I got lonely over time and decided to start dating. So I called up Ginny—one of the best moves I ever made—and

I said, "This is Bob." And she said, "Bob who?"

At any rate, "Bob Who" invited "Ginny Who" to the musical, "I Do, I Do," at the Chester Fritz Auditorium on the UND campus. I warned her that I'd have to take a couple of kids with me. "If you're going to date me," I said, "you're going to have to date a family, because that's what I am."

She agreed to go, and after the play we went back to my house where my housekeeper had fried up some hamburgers. The kitchen was covered in grease. The first thing Ginny did was to start wiping everything down. And I thought, well, this might turn out okay.

I told her what her ex-husband had said about her being a lush and she became indignant. It turned out she was a complete teetotaler and never drank at all. It was just another lie that some guys will make up to get somebody into bed.

We found out pretty quickly how much we had in common. She was the mother of four children and in the very same circumstances as I was. We talked a lot in those early days about what was important to each of us. We agreed that our kids were number one on the list. It wasn't long before I began to realize what a wonderful lady she was and how crazy her ex-husband was to have lost her.

As we became closer we wondered if our kids would get along with each other. So we rented a 25-foot camper, and I took my oldest daughter's VW Beetle and a tent, and we headed off to California for three weeks. We stopped at every national park there was and we camped and slept in the camper or in the tents. We did things as if we were one big family, which we were certainly heading toward. The kids seemed to enjoy that. We stopped in Yellowstone, Bryce Canyon, Virgin River. We went through Utah and to Las Vegas and we went into the Painted Desert in Arizona. We just had a ball. We had lots of rolls of quarters and every time we stopped at a gas station we gave each kid a quarter or two quarters so they could get a snack or a soda.

One of my daughter Barb's good friends brought along her boyfriend, Mike, on that trip. He had a driver's license and did some of the driving. Usually, when five o'clock rolled around, we let Mike drive the camper and Ginny and I went into the back and I had a cocktail. A couple of the girls thought I was an alcoholic and they poured out my bottle of booze, so that was the end of that. To this day that is a tale that always gets told at our family gatherings.

One day, as we were crossing South Dakota with Mike driving, he drifted across the center line a couple of times. A highway patrol car stopped us. The trooper came on as a real hard-nose and said to me, "You know, I can arrest every one of you here."

Then he asked me, "How many of you are there?" When I said there were 13, he looked into the camper at all of our faces and he kind of softened up. He said, "Well, I may not do it today." All in all, it was a very successful shake-down cruise for our two families who had meshed very quickly into one.

Not too long after that, I had to attend a meeting in Pierre, S.D. I said to Ginny, "Do you want to get hitched today?" One of the pilot trainers in UND's then-Center for Aerospace Sciences (CAS) flew us down to Pierre. Ironically, the plane belonged to Ginny's ex-husband who had bought it and leased it to CAS.

We got to the courthouse in Pierre at about 5 p.m. We didn't want an official, fancy wedding, because we needed to keep our expenses down, and God, we would have had to buy ten pairs of shoes. The justice of the peace was a very large man, at least 6'6", but his office was so tiny that not even our witnesses could get inside.

One of those trying to squeeze into the office was a tall guy by the name of Herbert Marshall. He was an Indian who was getting married right after us and he agreed to act as one of our official witnesses. The other witness was Jim Brosseau, whom I'd brought along to take pictures.

The JP came into the little office and he said, "Are you sure you folks want to do this?" We said yes, and he said, "Well then, you're married."

Afterward we went back to the small airport in Pierre and Mickey Knutson was there with some rice. It was so windy that when she threw the rice, it all blew away. We flew up to Minot and stayed in Mickey and Larry's house. Mickey went out and got some Champs Chicken and that was our wedding night. When we got back to Grand Forks, it turned out the kids knew all about our elopement and they tied a string of cans to the back of my car. And, with that, we were a family.

Ginny and I each sold our houses and we pooled our funds to build an 11-bedroom house on a lot I'd bought years earlier. Ginny drew up a sketch of what it would look like and we took it to an architect. Within two days they had it drafted out and a construction crew was digging the foundation. The house featured two wings of bedrooms that came together in a central family room with a 45-foot wide cathedral ceiling. There was a library that reached up three floors and a spiral staircase that led to the upper floors. The house had enough room for everybody, including private bathrooms. It had two propane furnaces two electric furnaces, two hot-water-heaters, two washers and two dryers.

Even though construction on our new home started immediately, progress on it began to slow down during that winter of 1974. Meanwhile, I had been in Bethesda, Md., helping the NIH develop a manual on new health professionals—nurse practitioners and physician assistants. I became aware of a program for the study of global health problems abroad, funded by the John E. Fogarty International Center, in partnership with the Fulbright program. Known as the Fogarty International Fellowship, it is closely allied with the NIH.

I applied and was awarded a three-month fellowship to study medical care in Norway, Sweden, Holland and Germany. I went over there in April and started in Norway. Ginny joined me in late April. Then, in early May when the kids got out of school they came over with Sue Dahlgren, who is now Sue Huus, my long-time assistant, and Ginny's mother, Jean Kieseau. I rented a Volkswagen camper and an Opal station wagon and we got a couple of tents and essentially camped out all over Europe. If you want something that forms up a family fast, try that. However, because of the noise level our brood generated, we got kicked out of just about every campground we checked into, and particularly in Germany.

But I do remember that during our visit to Holland, our Volkswagen camper broke down as we went across the Zuider Zee. I put all the kids in the back of the camper and pulled it into the closest campground we could find. They asked me how many we had, and I said, 13. They said, "Oh, we don't have enough room for that many." Then they asked me my name and I said, "Eelkema," and they said, "Oh, we'll give you two sites."

While I was married to my first wife, and shortly after the birth of our son, Robbie, I had a vasectomy. It seemed like the prudent thing to do at the time, perhaps even overdue, but when Ginny and I got married we talked about having a child of our own together. The vasectomy, however, seemingly made that impossible. Then I saw an article in the New York Times about a urologist at the University of California in San Francisco who did micro-surgery for kidney transplants. He also used the procedure to reverse vasectomies. I called him and found out he was booked solid for the next six months. Two weeks later he called. He'd had a cancellation, so I went out there. I had to be admitted to a hospital where I was given a low spinal. I found out I was his 38th patient. He had all of these doctors gathered around the operating table, staring at me. They were there because they wanted to learn the procedure, which would become very lucrative. Anyway, during the operation, this urologist put everything back together. At the crucial moment he yelled out, "I've got sperm!" Shortly after that I took Ginny with me to a meeting in Russia of the American College of Preventive Medicine. We saw the ballet and, later that night, we conceived our son, Rienk.

I think I experienced a renewal as a parent when Rienk was born. He readily bonded to both families, becoming the connecting link, the glue that held everything together.

Rienk was a balloon sculptor. He was a magician. He was a fourth-degree black belt in Tae Kwan Do. He was anything a kid would want to be. He was an Eagle Scout, Order of the Arrow. He was a counselor for two years at Camp Wilderness. He made his own uniforms. Rienk was a wonderful guy to go camping with because he knew everything. He was a kid you would want to have, a kid who was absolutely perfect.

He had an ability to relate to older people as well as younger. When we were in Disneyland there was a mother there with her crying kids. Rienk took out a balloon and made a hat, then a sword. Then he took some paper and did an origami. He knew about 450 origami things and he kept those kids from crying. It was amazing. He also taught self-defense to women. Another one of his students was a Navy seal, maybe twice his age. Rienk got him to quit smoking.

He was very much a peace-loving person who started training in Tae Kwan Do while still a child as a way of dealing with bullies. He was good kicker and earned a fourth-degree black belt early on. He eventually started his own Tae Kwan Do program at age 14. Teaching martial arts became his occupation when he got out of school. He'd attracted 120 students—including his wife-to-be—by the time he got married.

On his wedding day, all 10 kids, their wives and 12 grandchildren flew in from hither and yon to take part in the ceremony. Rienk had his nephew as the best man and he had one brother as a groomsman and all the other brothers as the ushers. The sisters were all involved in the whole thing as well.

He did an unheard-of thing when he invited Ginny and me to go along on his honeymoon to Disneyland in California. We went out there for three days and rode every ride in Disneyland with him. We were on Space Mountain four times one night. Rienk had to leave for home early because he was scheduled to give a black belt test in Bemidji, Minn., to one of his students at his Tae Kwan Do training academy. He kissed us both goodbye the night he left and we told him we loved him.

Rienk flew into Grand Forks and met up with the student and his family. They headed out toward Bemidji in separate cars. At about two o'clock that afternoon, as he was approaching Mentor, Minn., on a divided highway, he pulled out to pass a car ahead of him.

We found out later that only a few minutes earlier, an 85-year-old man living in a nearby assisted living nursing home had gotten into his car and headed west. He had passed the eye exam for his driver's license just a month earlier. Yet for some reason, in broad daylight, as the two-lane road he was traveling turned into a four-lane highway, he didn't see a single one of the 11 "Do not enter" signs that warned him to stay out of the eastbound lanes.

Without slowing down at all, he headed straight into the wrong lane. Rienk was just rounding a curve on that eastbound lane when the two cars hit head-on killing both of them. When we got the word we were absolutely numb. It was the worst experience I have ever had in my life, ever, ever, ever. Six days after his wedding, all of the family, the brothers and sisters and friends came back for the funeral. We had experienced the good times and the bad times all within a span of seven days.

It was absolutely devastating to Ginny and me. He was married for six days and on his way to making a living and doing his own thing. Every time I go by that crash site, I just cry.

I more or less quit working for a couple of years. I went into a deep, deep depression. I didn't give a damn about anything. I would go the medical meetings but I was filled with anger, and my attitude was, "The hell with everything."

I was living on the edge.

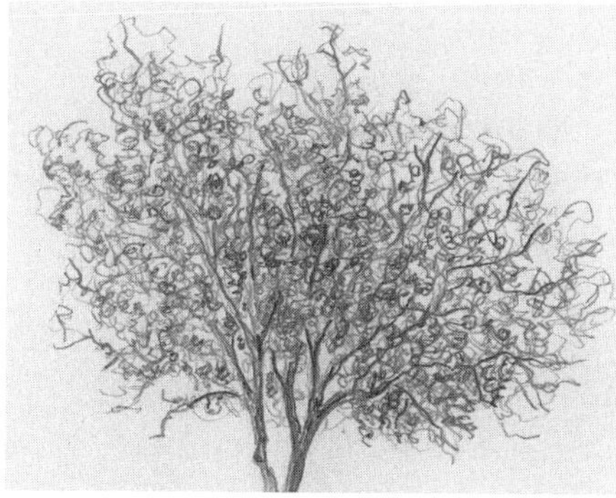

17

A Single Red Rose

FEBRUARY 25, 2000

IT IS 8:25 a.m., Mountain Time. I got up at 4 a.m. and got on the road by 4:30. I am nuttier than a fruitcake, I always have been, but I have to get down the road, you know. I stopped over at a club in Billings yesterday, where they have pari-mutuel betting. I bet a couple races and I made a little bit of money. So you can't take the bad ass out of me. I am still there.

I have taken the road from Billings and stopped at a Perkins restaurant in Bozeman for breakfast. Now I am going up towards the Big Sky Country. The Gallatin River is on my right and there are mountains on my left and right and it is a very curvy road. From Big Sky I am going to West Yellowstone and from West Yellowstone, I am heading over to Idaho and then down into Nevada. It is going to be a long day's drive. There are other roads to the west, I guess, that do go down there, but I would be going out of my way. This is the major highway through the Rocky Mountains. There was a little sun coming up this morning but it seems to have gone behind the clouds now. It is 31 degrees and a little bit overcast.

Yesterday I was in Circle, Mont., where I met with Patricia Wittkopp. Circle is a town of about 800 to 900 people. It is 75 miles from Sidney, 47 miles from Glendive and probably about 50 miles from Wolf Point. It is another 50 miles to Jordan. In other words, it is in the middle of absolutely nowhere. I remember the first time I came through here for a site visit, it was the middle of the night and I couldn't even see yard lights. Coming through here in the daylight, as I did yesterday, you see it is hilly country. You see an occasional ranch house. There are telephone lines or electric lines on the side of the road. The road is pretty rough, though. This is real lonesome country. I don't think that there is any doubt that Circle is the epitome of the rural health care dilemma in Montana. There isn't anything that is probably more rural.

I came over the top of a hill and I could see where every other little strip of land was summer fallow, with the hay in the middle. On the summer fallow land I could see a lot of snow, its white streaks interspersed with old hay land or old stubble. It was quite a beautiful sight, actually.

I got into Circle about 3 in the afternoon in drizzly rain. I could see by the signs that I was in McCone County, on the Red Water River. Another sign advertising the Travel Motel, called it "The best little snore house in town."

The first time I was here, I stayed at the Gladstone Hotel where the price was $10 a night without a bathroom and $20-a-night with a bathroom. I had to take the $10-a-night room because all the others were taken. I remember that night I had to prance down the hall to go to the bathroom, but that was my kind of hotel.

I stopped at the Wooden Nickel Café yesterday, where I'd arranged to meet Patricia. Inside, they had framed sacks for various different brands of potatoes. There were Hiawatha Washington Potatoes and Pennsylvania Pennywise brand. They had Fallon's brand, US #1, North Dakota Potatoes from Grafton, N.D. Those are the ones also known as Irish Eyes, US #1, Francis Fallon. They also had the Big Top Baker Potatoes from I don't know where in the heck. I think Idaho. Then they had some Western Montana

Potatoes, Dave Fischer Blue Hawk Russet Potatoes and AC Deuce Potatoes from Pasco, Wash. There was one from Big Buck Potatoes in Brill, Wis. How about that? And the special of the night was prime rib for $11.95, jumbo shrimp for $9.95.

Our interview was delightful. I learned that Patti's (everyone up here calls her Patti) husband, who she met at a rodeo, is a rancher, but something of an unwilling rancher. Apparently her husband's folks had moved into a nursing home and somebody had to come up and run the ranch. He and Patti moved up to Circle from Bozeman where Patti had graduated with a Bachelor of Science in Nursing degree. We always said that if we could get a nurse who is married to the local rancher, we would have the ideal person to provide health care in underserved areas. Boy, she really fits the specs.

We started out talking about the first time Mickey and I interviewed Patti and Dr. N.J. Hostettler, her preceptor, in 1989. He was really an interesting man. He was 66 years old, a native of Munich, Germany where he obtained his medical education. He served nine years, I think, in the German army, but he never could rise above private because one of his parents was born in San Francisco and evidently was Jewish. He migrated to the United States in 1951 and did some work in Chicago to get his internship and so forth. Then he worked in institutional settings to get his English sharpened up so he could pass the boards. He worked in Missouri, I think and then in Edgemont, S.D., for about a year. He moved up to Circle, Mont., in the U.S. Public Health Service. At the time we interviewed him he had been working as a doctor in Circle for 27 years.

I told Patti I had heard through the grapevine that Dr. Hostettler had suffered a stroke and wasn't in practice anymore.

"That's right," she said. "I am the only one here now."

"You are the sole provider for the area?"

"Yep. I get up and come to work and average between 28 and 35 patients a day."

In fact, she said, there were days where she'd see 60 patients and wouldn't get home until 11 p.m. Once a month a doctor comes up to review her charts.

Patti said she'd been looking for a long time for someone to fill in for her on a regular basis. As it is, she works pretty much 24/7. A physician assistant with 20 years' experience in the military called her recently from where he was working part time at a state prison. She invited him down and was impressed with his work and took him before the board that runs her clinic. They liked him as well and he is supposed to start soon.

Before she came to UND, Patti had been working with Dr. Hostettler for about 13 years as his office nurse. She was also the director of nursing at the local hospital and she helped in surgery. In 1988, the hospital was on the verge of closing. The administrator was a great visionary and thought the hospital could survive if it transformed itself into a Medical Assisted Facility, or MAF, where it could be staffed by medical extenders supervised by a physician—something like a Rural Health Clinic. She applied for a grant for a five-year pilot project but there was one thing missing from her application. There was no medical extender in the area to make the MAF feasible. She urged Patti to go back to school.

"And I said, 'Well, I don't think I can do it. I am already the public health nurse, the director of nursing, the doctor's right-hand man. I have a ranch and three kids.'"

Shortly after that she slipped on some ice while running to the post office and suffered a serious head injury.

"I ended up in the ICU and was laid up at home for three months," she said. "I couldn't do anything and it took me a long time to get back into shape. In those times, people would call me and ask how I could do all the things I'd been doing because it was taking two or three of them to do my job. But I realized that no one was expendable. So in August, when I started walking and then running to build up my strength, I just really felt that God was telling me to go back to school. So I got enough nerve up to call Mickey and she said, 'Oh yes, we are still looking for people.'"

Even then, she hesitated. "I dragged my feet doing all the preliminary paperwork and, by golly, Mickey called me one day and she said, 'Are you going to get through this or not? We want to send somebody down for a site visit and to interview you to see if you are what we want.' I told her about my concerns of having three kids who were 11, nine and five. She said 'Patti, if you don't go this year, you are not going to go because as soon as your daughter is a teenager, you are not going to be able to let her out of your sight. You are going to have to be there all the time.' And, you know, she was right. That was November and I started school in January."

I wasn't sure if she had ever seen the letter Dr. Hostettler wrote recommending her for the UND program and offering to be her preceptor. I'd brought it with me and took it out and read it to her. It is a classic.

> *"I was asked by our Director of Nurses, Mrs. Patti Wittkopp, if I would be willing to be her preceptor for training as a nurse practitioner. I am more than happy if I can be of help to Patti. I myself am 66 years old. I have practiced here in Circle for the past 27 years. I hope that I am able to continue practicing for a few more years yet. My son is in obstetrics in Pittsburgh, Pennsylvania and will not be coming back to Circle.*
>
> *I strongly believe that our small town and the small hospital have no attraction for a normal doctor, and only guys with problems of one kind or another will be candidates to succeed me. Therefore, I believe that the nurse practitioner/PA is the best solution to provide health care for the situation like ours here.*
>
> *Mrs. Wittkopp has worked here as a nurse for the past 12 years, the last four as our director of nurses. I have known Patti for all this time. She is conscientious, dependable, dedicated and trustworthy. I certainly have more confidence in being taken care of by Patti than by one of these characters that I have seen coming and going in and out of the small towns these days. Whatever I can do for Mrs. Wittkopp, to assist her in her goal to become a nurse practitioner, I will do. I have actually advised her and I have encouraged her to take this step.*
>
> *Sincerely,*
> *N. J. Hostettler, MD*

What a prophetic letter.

"Toward the end," Patti said, "he worked just on Tuesdays and Thursdays and the weekends because he kept a Saturday morning practice all these years. But he didn't see very many patients. He got down to where he was seeing, like, eight to 11 patients a week, and he told them 'Patti does all the work and I just take in all the money.' But, you know, he was there. I had a perfect arrangement. I really did.

"Doctor had a rough and gruff kind of exterior but, his heart and compassion was always there. When I first started he said, 'Well, I don't know how much I am going to be able to pay you because, you know, you will have to earn it.' Well, within the first three months, he had doubled my salary and he paid me very well. He was very generous to me. By the end he would say, 'You do all the work, Patti, you deserve it.'"

After Dr. Hostettler suffered a stroke, his wife took him back to Seattle where he had family. "She is so devoted to him. She never leaves his side, most of the time. He is in kind of a rehab center nursing home but they have moved him to a floor where he doesn't get a lot of rehab now, but his wife is just always there, after those nurses. She reviews the chart, she calls the doctors, she helps him eat and washes his clothes and she even presses all the pillowcases."

Patti was in Seattle a few months back for a PA conference and stopped by to visit Dr. Hostettler. "He had his eyes closed the whole time I was there and he just let me babble on and on and on," she said. "I told him all about the cows and you know this one and that one. He loves to gossip. So I was trying to think, well, what else can I tell Doctor? He just held my hand the entire time I was there and when I was done he said, 'Thank you, Patti, so much, for coming here.'"

When Patti graduated from UND in 1990 and came back to Circle, nurse practitioners and physician assistants were beginning to be accepted more and more in medical fields. Even so, proving herself to doctors remained a hurdle to be overcome.

"Getting physician acceptance was a challenge," she said. "It took me a while to build up a network. But I was lucky too because Doctor Hostettler had me go working with a group of cardiologists during my preceptorship and they became instrumental when I was first on my own. I could call them when I had a myocardial infarction or something. I could just get on the phone and call them and they knew if it was Patti calling, that they would take the patient. I never had to jump through the hoops much."

Still, she said, some physicians got nervous when they thought they were losing their patients to Patti, and they were reluctant to give her a lot of support.

"We had an older population of PAs in Montana because they were all military PAs or they were older and more experienced. And then we started getting these young ones coming in and working at the Billings Clinic. They didn't get a lot of respect. So when I would call up a doctor in the early years, I would say, 'This is Patti Wittkopp, I am a PA.' And they might say, 'What are you doing calling? Let me talk to your physician.' They didn't understand. So it took years of building up a rapport with them."

In the meantime, she said, the hardest part of her first year or so as a PA was in letting go of her old nursing role and stepping into a vastly different role with much more responsibility.

"I guess I went through a period, in that first year, where I said to myself, 'Why am I doing this? I can't do this.' I was really scared. But the second year it was more like, well, I can do this, this isn't so hard. I had a PA advisor, his name was Jim Reed. One day, he said, 'Never think you know it all. If you think you know it all, you don't know anything.' He said, 'Don't worry, if you are nervous about it, be glad that you are nervous about it because it means that you won't stop asking questions.' You know, that was real insightful because by the time I was into that second year where I said, oh, I guess I can do this, I started realizing that I needed a clear delineation of what I can do, what I can't do, and what I won't do to put myself in any kind of jeopardy. I had a real freedom from there on, knowing that I was just going to be able to do what I could do that day and take one patient at a time and then I was free of that."

At that point in our interview I wanted to go back to something Dr. Hostettler had said in his letter of recommendation. He'd mentioned outside doctors coming into small towns "with problems of one kind or another," and at one point referred to them as "characters." Was that just a generalization, I wondered, or did he have somebody in mind?

Patti then told me an amazing story about a "doctor" who worked at the hospital while she was a nurse. In fact, she was sure her accident on the ice was the result of being stressed out by this "doctor."

"I mean, he did surgery and it was so scary. He did, what was it, a hysterectomy, and I was the head scrub nurse. There was also an anesthesiologist, Dr. Rowe, who came up from Miles City. We still laugh about this because Dr. Rowe said, he didn't know me until that day. When I did my PA training I went down to Miles City and I worked with Dr. Rowe again. I walked into this surgical wing and he kept looking at me and looking at me and he said, 'I recognize your eyes. Only this time, they don't look like they are bugging out.' I was so stressed out. That doctor in Circle didn't know what he was doing. It was awful."

Not long after that she had her accident and was surprised when the doctor who had performed the hysterectomy visited her in the hospital. He brought her a single red rose and that was the last time anyone ever saw him. Not long after, it was determined that he was an imposter.

"I found out later that he disappeared the same day he brought me the flower. He must have stopped along the way and maybe he felt sorry for what he had done to me. So he gave me this red rose."

Can you imagine? This guy wasn't duly licensed or trained but he was willing to do a hysterectomy on a woman. My God, isn't that something? Those are the kinds of things you run into in a small hospital. It just boggles your mind that those kinds of things can happen.

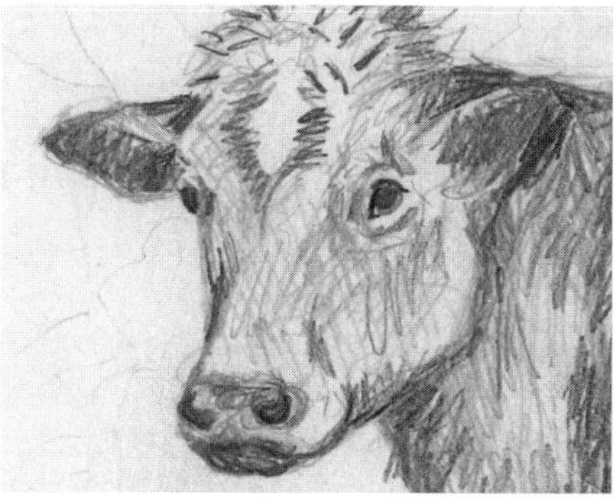

18

A Friend of No Man

IN 1990, JUST about the time Patti Wittkopp was heading back to Circle, Mont., to start her new career as a physician assistant, our program underwent some significant changes. Essentially, we lost all our funding—which is about as significant as you can get. At the same moment, for the first time since we'd been operating the program in 1972, we got more applications from prospective students than we had slots to fill.

I attribute that to the critical mass of NPs and PAs that UND and other schools had graduated and sent into the field. I've always thought our best recruiters were the graduates themselves. And, of course, the more medical extenders there were, the more doctors and nurses got used to the idea and even started relying on these odd medical hybrids to lift the burden from their shoulders.

There was one other big change that had been brewing for some time and which still bothers the daylights out of me. It's what led to the loss of our funding from both the Kellogg Foundation and the NIH Division of Health Manpower, and changed the emphasis of our training.

Initially, we were both a nurse practitioner and a physician assistant program, and were accredited by the national organizations of both groups. But in 1990 the American Nurses Association (ANA) withdrew their support of our program. They were unhappy that we were training nurses who had not earned either a baccalaureate or a master's degree. That was largely true—although there were a few, here and there, who did enter the program with advanced degrees.

Still, in the 1970s and '80s, many nursing schools—including the one in Grand Forks at St. Michael's Hospital—were only two-year programs. If we had held out all those years for four-year graduates or master's-degreed nurses, we wouldn't have been able to find enough people to train. And we would have denied advanced training to quite a few, very qualified people.

In my experience, the nurses we trained who had come from a two-year program were very capable and professional. After our first MEDEX years, all our students came from an environment where they'd been working as nurses in rural areas and gaining in experience whatever they might have lacked for want of a college degree. Personally, I don't think any of them lacked anything.

But there was a movement afoot within nursing organizations that was shifting the focus from the practical to the academic. When the ANA withdrew support, the Kellogg Foundation followed, as it too was coming around to the idea of "better educated" nurses.

The biggest criticism I would have from what I have seen today is that they have a lot of very theory-driven master's programs in PA and NP programs which have nothing to do with the real world of medicine. It seemed to me that the nursing world got into a situation where they felt like the only way they could get respect from doctors was to add all these academic programs, which I think miss the point of nursing altogether.

What they are saying is that if you have a master's degree it gives you a little bit more clout in the working world. I don't think it means anything more than that. I don't think master's-educated nurses are any better than the ones who have an associate degree. I'm going on a bit of a rant here, but I think that behind the push for a master's education you will find that universities are the institutions ultimately profiting from that whole push. The people who are providing the services and the people who are receiving the services don't benefit, whether you have a master's or Bachelor of Science in Nursing or just a plain old associate's degree.

Out of that movement toward academic credentials the federal government found reasons not to fund us. We had to change quickly otherwise we were going to lose the whole program. We'd already increased our student-load from 30 to 60 in 1989 and in 1990 boosted it to 80—the number of seats we had in our lecture hall.

In order for us to maintain our economic viability, we funded the program from that point on completely by student tuition. Again, thanks to Tom Clifford's support as president, we were able to put 100 percent of that tuition into the program.

Meanwhile, we still had the blessing of the physician assistant organizations, so we dropped the NP element and went total PA. We still only accepted nurses and for the next ten years we trained and graduated some 804 physician assistants.

In the beginning we had some pretty motivated students who did well on their national exams. We had a 98 percent pass-rate. When we increased our numbers to 80 students, however, we kind of fell down. Our faculty—which we recruited from local physicians—wasn't ready for the increased load. This was a big change and it was very difficult for them to handle. But with persistence and a commitment to staying the course, we were able to show we could do just as well with 80 as 30. The faculty became accustomed to it and student scores rose once again.

When I retired in 2000, I was interviewed by some UND people who were putting together a videotape summarizing my career. It was shown at my retirement dinner and it had me talking about the INMED Program, the expansion of the medical school, the MEDEX Program, nurse practitioners and physician assistants and so forth. But one job that I mentioned during that interview was cut out. I'd even told the people making the tape that it was probably the most significant accomplishment in my life. For some reason they didn't think it was important. I couldn't help feeling then, as I still do today, that the reason it was discounted had to do with the topic: the mentally retarded.

Let me back up a bit, a good bit, in fact. In 1903 the state legislature approved funding for the construction of a home for the retarded in Grafton. This "Institution for the Feeble Minded" opened in 1904 and, thereafter, the mentally retarded were sent there rather than being mixed in with the population at the state "hospital for the insane" in Jamestown. In spite of the archaic and degrading terms "feeble minded" and "insane," the Grafton facility in some ways described social progress. Until then, anyone in North Dakota with any kind of mental disability was simply considered to be crazy.

In the 1930s the "feeble minded" appellation was discarded in favor of a new name: The Grafton State School. By the mid-1950s, the school was becoming overcrowded. In 1957 a non-profit organization called the Association for Retarded Citizens (ARC) incorporated itself in North Dakota to monitor the problem. In the early 1960s, the state converted the former San Haven tuberculosis sanitarium, not far from Grafton, as a satellite hospital. Together, at their peak, the two institutions housed about 1,300 residents.

With the institution of the Community Mental Health Center Act under the Kennedy Administration in the early 1960s, a massive deinstitutionalizing of state hospitals and state schools swept the country. The populations of those facilities fell as funds were made available to local communities for the care of what was becoming known as the "developmentally disabled." But not everyone was treated locally and, in time, the enthusiasm and funding for community-based centers waned. In North Dakota, the Grafton and Dunseith facilities continued housing the mentally disabled and, once again, overcrowding became an issue.

Predictably, in a conservative state known for its parsimonious response to the needs of the disenfranchised, the two aging facilities fell into gross disrepair on the outside, while care within the walls became chaotic at best and non-existent at worst. So much so that, in 1980, the ARC brought suit in federal district court against the state. It charged that North Dakota had failed to perform its duty. State law required providing the developmentally disabled with services aimed at lifting them to the fullest extent of their potential—but in a setting that was least likely to abridge their personal liberties. Specifically, on behalf of six mentally retarded citizens, the ARC condemned the treatment and inhospitable surroundings of the Grafton and Dunseith sites.

In the fall of 1981, North Dakota District Court Judge Bruce Van Sickle issued a federal court order that the state immediately begin resolving the deficiencies at Grafton and Dunseith. Van Sickle decided to appoint a court observer to monitor the state's progress or lack thereof in responding to his order.

Ed Klecker, who worked in the department, wrote out a proposal suggesting that the UND Department of Community Medicine provide the monitor for the job. He walked over to the judge's house and presented it to him. Shortly afterward, I got a note on my desk saying that Judge Van Sickle wanted to see me. The long and the short of it is that I was appointed the monitor and remained in that job until April 1991.

No sooner had I been appointed, however, than the plaintiff's attorney objected. So the judge set up a hearing which I attended along with representatives of the state and ARC. At that meeting, Judge Van Sickle told everyone that he had gone out and talked to doctors around the state about me, and had talked to my staff and had even talked to officials at UND.

What he said next should have shocked me, I suppose, but I took it as a compliment. Addressing himself to me, he said, "You tend to be a procrastinator and the doctors out there don't necessarily like you. But you have a good staff. And, you know, the person I hire has got to be a friend of no man. And you, Dr. Eelkema, most certainly qualify."

I thought that was a backhanded compliment because I laughed quite heartily. What he was really saying, in his legalistic way, was that I wasn't in anybody's back pocket. I was my own man and I wouldn't be in the back pocket of either the plaintiff or the defense, nor would I be playing any games. I considered it the ultimate compliment. That is the way I have been most of my life. I'm a friend of no man. I call them as I see them. I've been known to be just a little bit short with people, yes. But there's an awful lot that got accomplished. I could probably adopt the theme song, "I Did It My Way," by Frank Sinatra.

I immediately hired a staff and, although I remained on the hot seat for that job, our people—Mickey Knutson, Dr. Bud Shutt, Ed Klecker, Jack Brookes and Kari Conrad—did an exemplary job. I think that we helped nudge the state toward providing better services to the developmentally disabled, unfortunate souls who were pretty much pushed into a back room and forgotten. But, politically, it was very unpopular. We got everybody pissed off at us. You know, the way I saw it, our job was to afflict the comfortable instead of comforting the afflicted. I really enjoyed doing that. It seems like I got myself in a wringer all the time. My name was in the paper most of the time and we were the brunt of quite a few personal attacks. But, it was worth everything. I will never regret it.

I got a nice letter from Judge Bruce Van Sickle applauding me for my activities as they related to improving the welfare of people who couldn't really speak for themselves. We affected the lives of those people over ten years, making sure the judge's decree was followed by the state. It was kind of a thankless job, but I felt like I was really doing something worthwhile for some of the lesser endowed citizens of the state. And that, I think, was the job in which I took the most gratification.

When I retired in 2000 at the age of 70, our program had four applicants for every slot, and we had 80 slots. We had a reputation par excellence throughout the country. In all, we had graduated more than 1,100, with a very high percentage of them practicing in rural and underserved areas. We didn't build a lot of brick and mortar. But we deployed a lot of people in areas of need where they were affecting lives of hundreds of thousands of people.

Eventually, Tom Clifford retired as president of UND. New presidents and new deans took over, people who weren't from

North Dakota and who had little appreciation of the need for rural medical care and of how we were quite efficiently filling that need. About a year before I retired, the new president was under pressure to cut the budget. The new medical school dean was asked to decide what three programs were expendable. He was given an hour to make the decision and he put the PA Program on the expendable list, even though it was self-supporting, we brought in outside students, we were in the black financially and we had always supported the medical school. He decided the PA Program was not the major mission of the medical school and would have to be put on the block.

Fortunately, we got a lot of support from outside organizations. We got some support from the State Board of Higher Education and we got some support from the Association of Physician Assistants within the state. The dean backed off, but it left a bad taste in my mouth to think that we were almost sold down the drain without our knowledge.

As long as I was chairman and as long as I was there, they didn't interfere any further. A year before I retired, my friend and colleague Dr. Jim Brosseau, one of the most respected doctors in the state, took over the Department of Community Medicine as chairman. Years before that, I'd sent him away to get his master's degree in public health. In the very early years he was co-director of our program. He was also one of our faculty members and just a great help.

Jim is one of the kindest people I've ever known. He was thoroughly capable of running a department in a medical school, but his personality didn't have the "friend of no man" sandpaper that mine did. The academic world is such that you really have to stand up to a lot of people who, while super-sophisticated, are just not very nice. The infighting that goes on in academia can be cold and vicious. I felt bad that Jim walked into almost an ambush when he took over. When I left, there was no one there to defend the program the way I did, essentially by being a little bit abrasive when needed. There isn't an abrasive bone in Jim's body, but what a smart man he is.

He brought in two-top level physicians to the program—one from public health, the other from the EIS. They were superb teachers who brought in a lot of grant money. But when the largest of those grants arrived, the dean took half of it and gave it to a different department. Appalled, both of those doctors eventually left. One became the chief health officer in Michigan and the other the chief health officer in Montana. That's the caliber of people Jim recruited.

But the dean did everything to undercut his activity and to take advantage of him. Really, the straw that broke the camel's back was when the dean dissolved the Department of Community Medicine and put it into the Department of Family Medicine and then left town on a business trip. Now, the chairman of family practice is a perfectly capable guy, but he has no experience in biostatistics and epidemiology. He never went through a school of public health. He doesn't know what he doesn't know.

Jim didn't realize you had to fight sometimes unfairly, which I did during the whole time I was chairman. There was always somebody who wanted to take my role away or was jealous of what I was doing. One thing is certain: they didn't like the money that we were bringing in. They thought it should have been distributed to the university as a whole. I just went ahead and decided that was money to develop the new health practitioner, not to increase research funding for basic science.

Disgusted with the way things turned out, Jim left the university he'd been proud of and had worked so hard for all his professional life. He now practices internal medicine in Grand Forks. He's my private doc, in fact. And he'll always be my friend. He is just a loyal, loyal stand-up guy.

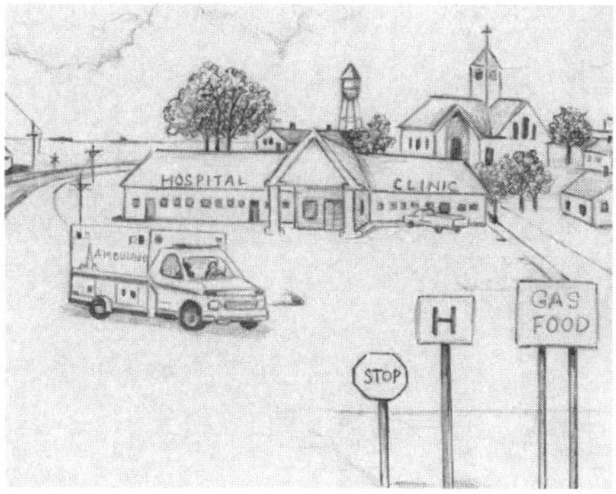

19

Letting Go (More or Less)

I THINK YOU'LL find that most doctors who have any experience working in an emergency room earned that experience early in their careers as a young med student, intern or resident. Unless one actually chooses emergency medicine as a specialty, I think it's safe to say that most doctors are not unhappy to leave behind the often chaotic pace of the ER for their chosen field.

When I was a young doctor, my emergency rooms were in Seattle hospitals through the University of Washington and, again, during my hitch in the uniformed health services in the Navajo country of Arizona and New Mexico and then in Berkeley during the final year of my training for a Master in Public Health degree. At the age of 70, an age at which many doctors retire or have long since retired, I decided to become an emergency room physician once more.

As with many physicians, medicine wasn't simply a job or a career to me; it was a calling—which is why I just couldn't stay retired. Nor could I remain paralyzed by grief over the death of my son. Friends and colleagues had tried to console me for many months, but I couldn't or wouldn't allow them to break through that hard shell of heartache. Ultimately, it was an old medical school colleague named Lowell Mickelson who broke through my defenses with the offer of a job as a fill-in doc at small-town emergency rooms. Clearly, it was time for this physician to heal himself.

Mick, as I called him, had a company that provided doctors to small-town hospitals in North Dakota and Minnesota. I was available for two weekdays and most weekends, and usually worked from 25 to 30 hours. I'd get up at 2 a.m. in Grand Forks to get to a noon appointment in places like Rolla or Cooperstown in North Dakota, or Bagley and Mahnomen in Minnesota. Very often I had to drive through snow and sleet, but I was very seldom late. In all, I spent about nine years working for Mick and put 50,000 miles a year on my truck.

For the most part I enjoyed it. I think the most satisfying work I did was at the hospital in Mahnomen, Minn., about 80 miles southeast of Grand Forks. It's one of a handful of U.S. cities located completely on an Indian reservation—in this case the Chippewa's White Earth Reservation. The nurses were quite grateful I was there. At the beginning, there was a second physician in the ER with a couple more who came in later. I was actually elected the physician director and even got my picture and name on the wall.

Unfortunately, Mick contracted non-Hodgkin's lymphoma and died prematurely. I lost not only an advocate but a good friend. A problem when you grow older is that all your friends or colleagues have either retired or died and your references have gone down the tube. And when you're working alone or with only one or two other docs, it's hard to get work at another ER if you don't have a good reference.

Mick's company, in the meantime, was growing and had people working in the front office who weren't physician-trained. If I had any problems with hospital administrators or nurses, I no longer had someone who knew me and who could vouch for me.

Meanwhile, at the hospitals themselves, I saw administrators come and go in a constant flow. I realized that nothing and no one is ever permanent in a small-town hospital. There was always some kind of musical chairs going on. I think it's because no one can make a silk purse out of a sow's ear. Unfortunately, as small hospitals go, they're always financially strapped. They are always looking for ways to make some money and sometimes your job is in jeopardy because of a change in administration where the new CEO doesn't know anything about you.

A lot of times the only way a small hospital can make it is to sell out to bigger clinics. And that's what happened to Mahnomen. They sold out to a bigger clinic in Fargo which put their own people up there. So that job kind of melted away.

In medicine there sometimes is an attitude that bigger is better—bigger hospitals, bigger departments, bigger practices with more doctors. There's no question that when it comes to an emergency room, the bigger the budget, the bigger array of lifesaving equipment you have on hand. But usually the budget isn't so big in small towns, and often the array of equipment begins and ends with a helicopter ride to a bigger town with a bigger hospital.

Of course, the bigger the ER, it seems, the longer a patient has to wait to be seen. That is one thing I do like about the small town ER. So many of them put out a little sign in the waiting room that says if you haven't been seen in 10 minutes come on up and see the receptionist. In those ERs, we never let a patient sit for very long. I liked that. In that case, people get pretty damn good care. What small hospitals lack in technology they make up for in humanity and personal caring. It really does make a difference.

I didn't work for long after Mick died. In fact, I'd describe my work after Mick's death as walking on eggs. I was always afraid I was going to crack one. For a time I did work up in Roseau and Baudette in northern Minnesota. When I went up to Roseau they had my birthdate and my age right there in the clinic in front of the nurses. So, even though I may not have looked 80, they knew that I was 80. So any little stumble or any little mistake was scrutinized to a greater degree. And I always felt like I was under a microscope. It wasn't pleasant. I worked in a place once where the other doctor called me "the old man." He was a young doctor. And

I think, when you're young, anyone who is 20 years older is the old man. I felt kind of intimidated by it.

Of course, working in an ER you have to be mindful and subservient to a wide variety of constituencies. Probably the most important are the nurses who can make or break you. Some are very grateful that you're there. Others are looking at you with a great deal of scrutiny and see defects and the possibility of aging getting the best of you.

After being sent to several hospitals I hadn't seen before, I made it a point to start looking at a hospital's availability of decent housing or a place to sleep while on call. I wanted, at least, a room with an open window. There was one hospital where the on-call room had only a skylight. It was a fire hazard; in an emergency, you couldn't get out of the place. One hospital's on-call room was on the second floor right next to the patients. And I had to walk down that long hall right past them to take a shower or use the rest room. Sometimes after a long day I looked like the wreck of the Hesperus. And walking all the way down those halls and back, it just made me feel uncomfortable.

I think one of the hardest things about those small-town ER jobs was the feeling of being very alone. You're not just the only doctor in the ER, most of the time you're the only doctor within miles. Whatever came in, you had to handle it. During my time in Mahnomen it wasn't uncommon to have multiple car accidents in the winter—lots of people coming in with severe injuries. Way out there, in the middle of an ice storm, you just don't have the availability of ambulances or helicopters to transfer patients. You just have to do the best you can.

There were a few very tight situations. I've had people come in with foreign bodies in their eyes. And I've tried to get an ophthalmologist to come out to see them. But those docs went into ophthalmology so they wouldn't have to be on call late at night. And, like a lot of specialists, they very rarely come out to see a patient. It's almost impossible to rouse them. A couple of times I had to insert a chest tube in a patient who was coding. I did it at the direction of an ER doc in Fargo, speaking over the phone with me. It could get a little bit on the scary side.

I worked a few times in Park Rapids, Minn., near Cass Lake where Ginny and I have a summer home. That service got to be very heavy, especially in the summer with a lot of tourists at the lake. Whenever I was at an ER close to a reservation I saw an awful lot of diabetes and an awful lot of people who didn't take care of themselves. They were overweight and obese, and they came in with insulin shock or in a coma.

Most people who come into small-town ERs are usually people without insurance and the hospitals have to take care of them. They over-smoke, over-eat, over-drink, and you are trying to keep them from dying prematurely from their own excesses. It was frustrating. Once I had a 400 pound, 50-year-old male come in with a stroke. And his son asked me, "What are you going to do to get him better?" Pretty soon you get hardened to it. But I could never feel much self-fulfillment treating such cases. To have people only coming in when there was a crisis really is a failure of medicine.

One other thing you get used to or hardened by is the idea that not everything a patient tells you is the gospel truth. So many people play cat-and-mouse with you. I've seen patients who have had coronary bypass and stents put in, but they come into the ER and say they've never had any problems at all. Unless you've got the medical record in front of you, you have to take them at their word.

Often we would see patients who had spent months or years being treated in large, big-city cancer clinics. They'd gone through the entire oncology system and had finally been sent home. Then, when their condition ultimately deteriorated, we would see them in the local ER. Usually we had no information about their medical history. We would talk to the relatives and eventually it would become clear that this was a terminal patient. It sometimes got very emotional.

After about a year I decided the miles I was driving every week, the feeling of being scrutinized at every turn, the inhospitable conditions—pun intended—I often worked in, and that uncomfortable feeling of being alone took its toll. This time when I retired there was no video celebrating my life, no fancy dinner, no speeches. On the other hand, this time retirement was completely my idea. It was just time to let go.

During those ten years on the road I kept a small tape-recorder by my side in the truck. I'd fill up cassettes with ideas, anecdotes, lessons learned and just odd thoughts and commentary about life in general. Sometimes I would send them off to my kids or friends. Not long after I retired I took some time to jot down what I guess you would call my philosophy of life as captured on those cassettes. These ideas aren't lofty or theoretical aphorisms of the Kahlil Gibran type. They're more like battle-tested observations and conclusions about navigating a survivable course from the seas of today to the shores of tomorrow.

Here, then, in no particular order, or even logic, is the "why" behind my "who."

- Never advertise what you are going to do. A lot of times you just don't live up to the expectations.
- People in trouble do not need more trouble. It is better to be of help and solace than to be retributive and critical.
- Every individual has a blind spot, including myself. It is my hope that I can know this in myself and understand it in others.
- When very frustrated about some wrong inflicted on you or upon society, sit down and write a scathing letter to the inflictor of the pain. It will do wonders for your mental health. Just be sure you don't mail it.
- I used to write really harsh letters-to-the-editor about things I felt were wrong or unjust, but I never actually sent them. Whatever it was, I got over it. I've learned there are always two sides to a story, sometimes three. There's my side, your side and sometimes a middle-ground side. Usually, nobody's totally right or totally wrong. There are many shades of gray in this world.

- Don't confuse an education with being educated. No matter what school you went to, or what degrees you've earned, you're not educated until you recognize you don't know everything.
- A crisis can create greater understanding and wisdom. Sometimes a single failure creates more growth than a constant series of successes.
- Don't let rejection become an obstacle. During virtually every project I have done in life, I have been rejected. But I believed in what I was doing, I trusted my judgment and I persisted. Because of that approach, I have been labeled by some as stubborn and unmanageable. Sometimes those are good qualities.
- I have lived long enough to see my grandson take over the family farm and do well. I lost a son, but also a son-in-law, Harold Helm, one of the greatest guys I've ever met. He died of pancreatic cancer. Everybody has pain and suffers through tragedies, large and small. They make you humble and a little bit more empathetic to the trials of others. Nobody gets through life without pain. It's whether or not you allow it to change you for the better that's important.
- Don't let the performance of a good deed hang on the possibility of recognition or reward. A good deed performed with an ulterior motive is just a deed.
- To be trusted, you must be trustworthy. That is no easy thing in a world set up to believe that what you are worth determines whether or not you are worthy.
- Every person should be encouraged and allowed to take risks. This is sometimes the most difficult precept for a parent, especially a parent of a disabled child.
- There are very few people in this world who see a situation that needs to be rectified and rectify it. Most people go with the flow.

- Everybody should have an animal. They like you regardless of what you do and they seldom take retribution. When you come home they're excited about seeing you again.
- You never get anything unless you ask for it.

One thing I've gleaned from the field of medicine that applies to daily life is that if you want to effect change and see something happen, it takes a long time. In fact, it takes the patience of Job. In a sense, our training program at UND really revolutionized the practice of medicine. That there's going to be a team approach to practicing medicine—doctors, nurses, PAs, NPs, occupational therapists, physical therapists and pharmacists working as a cohesive unit—is not just a foregone conclusion. That change is already under way because there just aren't enough first-line doctors to answer the needs of all those areas crying for primary care. It is exciting to know that we were among the pioneers.

One item I have only recently come to appreciate: As you grow older you realize the importance of friendship and in maintaining friendships. When friends die it is a difficult, difficult issue. Even though I lost Dr. Shutt as a good friend, before he died I called him every other day and we had wonderful conversations. As my friends gradually fall by the wayside, I notice that I have become extremely good friends with my family. My daughters and my sons have become my companions, my sounding boards and the people that I talk to most frequently. We talk, we write, and we travel together. I enjoy them just tremendously. Plus, my wife Ginny, a wonderful woman, is my best friend. That is the essence of being mentally healthy.

Finally, we were always taught in medical school that we should not present ourselves as proficient with any treatment or procedure that was superior to one that's generally being done. I realize some doctors are better than others, but it's not advertising that makes them better. Andy Rooney once put it this way, "If it's advertised I'm not using it."

Boy, I believe in that one—because, that's who I am. And by now, you know why.

Acknowledgements

NO WORTHWHILE EFFORT becomes reality as a result of one man's labors. So it is with the program that trained and graduated more than 1100 nurse practitioners and physician assistants between 1971 and 2000 through the Department of Community Medicine at the University of North Dakota School of Medicine and Health Sciences.

The number of dedicated individuals who helped make health care more accessible to citizens of rural, out-of-the-way communities through this program is long and impressive. This book is dedicated to the graduates of that pioneering program—the ones who went forth and used their skills to help those in need. But without a sense of duty brought to the task of creating a workable, sustainable program from scratch, there would be no story to tell.

I am especially indebted to the following individuals who believed in what we were doing and, in a time of great debate over the role of doctors and the future of health care delivery, made believers of just about everyone. One has only to step into any emergency room in the country to find capable and quite professional nurse practitioners and physician assistants whose medical skills and careers were made possible by a handful of early training programs that challenged the status quo and revolutionized medicine through a new breed of health care providers.

At the head of the list is a man named **Tom Clifford**. I can't say enough about Tom, the president of the University of North Dakota during our first 20 years. At risk to his own reputation, Tom supported our efforts when others in the university complained about the way we operated. We were really an experimental program. But Tom allowed us to expand as we saw fit. He didn't just do that for us. That was his standard operating procedure with anyone who had a good idea and demonstrated the will to make it happen. He would give you his support and give you plenty of room to succeed—or fail. The catch was, if you didn't deliver, Tom had no qualms about showing you the door. If I hadn't had Tom Clifford at the top during these years, I'm sure I would have been wiped out. If you don't have support at the top you might as well get out.

Another person to whom I owe a large debt is **Dr. Jim Brosseau**, a homegrown graduate of the UND School of Medicine. He became assistant director of the MEDEX Program and added a tremendous amount to the program. Jim was an excellent teacher in the department and a loyal colleague. He took over the Department of Community Medicine as chair a year before I left. Today Jim is one of the most respected and popular internists in North Dakota. Borrowing from that old Sara Lee bakery goods jingle: Nobody doesn't like Jim Brosseau. He's my private doctor in Grand Forks and he'll always be my friend.

When I first came to the university in 1964, **Mickey Knutson**, a faculty member in the UND College of Nursing, was an immediate help and support. Together we developed a program that added senior nursing students to the class in epidemiology that I was teaching to sophomore medical school students. Mickey then joined the Department of Community Medicine and she and I were pretty much joined at the hip for the next 20 years. We were both committed to training nurse practitioners and physician assistants. Mickey was an excellent listener which made her a wonderful counselor for our students. She had all the necessary qualities of insight, wisdom and understanding. It was Mickey who suggested we draw on the pool of local nurses as prospective students in our PA and NP program. She and **Judy DeMers**, who also came to the department from the nursing school were invaluable in their commitment and expertise. Later, Mickey convinced **Barbara Lee** of the Kellogg Foundation of the value of our program. We were subsequently funded quite liberally from Kellogg over a period of many years.

One thing that was really important to making the program work was the loyalty of **Sue Huus**. I hired her when her name was Dahlgren, before she married Bob Huus. She stayed with me as a capable and hard-working administrative assistant and supportive colleague the entire time I was at UND. She later continued to work with Jim Brosseau when he took over the department. She is a wonderful lady.

A couple who really made life easier for me was **Martha Adams** and her husband, **Billy**. I met Martha when she was a public health nurse in Omaha, Neb. I later convinced her to join the department at UND. She suffered from diabetes from the age of 15 and had tremendous problems with it all of her life. She developed small angle glaucoma and ended up blind. Even then, she went to the University of Colorado and graduated magna cum laude in community health nursing. Billy was our computer specialist. Martha sent me a wonderful letter after my son, Rienk, died. When I was really grieving I'd pick Martha up and we'd go for a drive. What a tremendous support she was during that time. Diabetes finally took her. Only about a six months year later, Billy died of a stroke. They were just an ideal couple.

There were many people in the department who became friends over the years and who were loyal and pleasant to work with. If a person couldn't laugh I really didn't care about working with them. They had to be transparent and honest. Also, in any organization, the most important people are the ones who interact with the public, either in the office or on the phone. So we were very fortunate to have competent and friendly staffers including **Avis Reynolds**, who was with us from age 17, **Karen Allard**, **Ruth Kalenze**, **Rhonda McDaniel**, **Terry Lang**, **Annette Larson**, **Dawn Lykken**, **Melissa Gardner**, **Condetta Ness**, **Linda Huss**, **Marge Winbourn**, **Suzanne Corbett**, **Bill Sturm**, **Sandy Tebben** and **Terrie Jo Wold**. There may be others, living and dead, who should be mentioned but whom I cannot recall. To you, I extend my apologies.

It was while studying for my Master in Public Health degree at Berkeley that I became best friends with a fellow student, **Dr. Bud Shutt**. He was a very intelligent man. After Berkeley he became chief health officer in Bangkok and contributed to health policy in Vietnam. After he opened up the Medical School of the Nile in Egypt, he was looking for his next assignment. I made him the chairman of the international division and co-director of the PA Program. He was very much into training PAs and was a superb doctor.

Of course, without the encouragement of **Dr. Dick Smith**, whom I'd met at the University of Washington during my residency training in epidemiology, the program at UND might never have existed. It was Dick who originally introduced me to the MEDEX concept in 1969, and without a doubt it was Dick who changed my life more than anybody. He was definitely my mentor, advocate and cheerleader. He was very helpful in opening doors for us in Washington and in developing our first MEDEX curriculum.

Not long after I'd spoken to Dick about MEDEX, Judy DeMers and I went out to Seattle and, within two to three weeks, put together an application to become one of the first MEDEX schools in the nation. Then Dick pointed us to the office of **Paul Sanazaro** of NIH's Division of Health Manpower Research, where I personally hand-delivered our proposal. Much of our early funding came from Sanazaro's office, with the help of one of his key assistants, **Doug Fenderson**, a North Dakota native who understood our mission and believed in it from the start. Once we'd won our grant, we needed to find a faculty to teach the courses and preceptors to mentor our students. Among those who did yeoman's work in rounding up prospective physicians was **Dr. Willard Wright**.

Later, Dick Smith got us involved in a program that sought to transfer the technical capabilities of training PAs to Third World countries. In that respect, I hired **Ed Klecker**, who provided welcome support. Subsequently, our staff had an opportunity to work overseas. Mickey went to Lesotho, in south Africa. **Bonnie Bata** and a few other staff people worked in Guyana. I, myself, went with Dick Smith to Liberia to try and get a program started. Other people in the program had been available for Pakistan and the Marshall Islands. It was very much a learning experience and very exciting.

Some of them still toil on, others are gone. But I still see their faces and feel their spirit and wonder at the deeds we all accomplished with little fanfare but a healthy measure of satisfaction.

I want to thank my son, Robbie Eelkema, for his tireless work as a foot-leather soldier to make this book a reality.

—ROBERT EELKEMA, M.D.,
Grand Forks, North Dakota, 2012

"Life Lessons, According to Dave"

Feel your feelings fully

Be honest

Keep your promises

Live fully

Love wastefully

Be your own person

Index

About the Author

DR. ROBERT EELKEMA'S dedication to improving public health began early in his career. After completing his medical training, he joined the Epidemiological Intelligence Service of the Centers for Disease Control, the organization credited with stamping out small pox as a worldwide disease. He participated in the EIS efforts to understand and eradicate polio which posed a serious threat to public health in the 1950s.

In 1964, Dr. Eelkema accepted his first academic appointment in the Department of Physiology at the University of North Dakota School of Medicine and Health Sciences, and served as physician in the UND Student Health Service. Four years later, he was appointed chairman of the newly created Department of Community Medicine at the UND medical school.

During his nearly 40-year career at UND, he was a key leader in transforming the then-two-year basic sciences program into a full, four-year, MD degree-granting medical school. He served as chairman of school's Medical Affairs Committee, working with the state's physicians and national granting agencies to build political and fiscal support for the four-year medical school. After the medical education program was approved by the North Dakota legislature in 1973, Dr. Eelkema served as chairman of the Medical Operations Committee at UND.

In addition to his leadership in initiating the MEDEX and Physician Assistant/Nurse Practitioner programs at UND, he was instrumental in developing the Indians into Medicine (INMED) Program to attract American Indians to the field of health care.

Dr. Eelkema is also known for spearheading the state's effort to deinstitutionalize the developmentally-delayed residents of the Grafton State School in Grafton, ND, and a similar state-sponsored facility at Dunseith, ND—a process that proved to be both controversial and contentious.